Manual of Practical Gynecological Oncology

Manual of Practical Gynecological Oncology

Edited by

Basil Bloch, Katrien Dehaeck and Robbert Soeters

Gynecologic Oncology Unit, Department of Obstetrics and Gynecology, University of Cape Town and Groote Schuur Hospital, Cape Town, South Africa

CHAPMAN & HALL MEDICAL

London · Glasgow · Weinheim · New York · Tokyo · Melbourne · Madras

Published by Chapman & Hall, 2–6 Boundary Row, London SE1 8HN, UK

Chapman & Hall, 2–6 Boundary Row, London SE1 8HN, UK

Blackie Academic & Professional, Wester Cleddens Road, Bishopbriggs, Glasgow G64 2NZ, UK

Chapman & Hall GmbH, Pappelallee 3, 69469 Weinheim, Germany

Chapman & Hall USA, One Penn Plaza, 41st Floor, New York NY 10119, USA

Chapman & Hall Japan, ITP-Japan, Kyowa Building, 3F, 2-2-1 Hirakawacho, Chiyoda-ku, Tokyo 102, Japan

Chapman & Hall Australia, Thomas Nelson Australia, 102 Dodds Street, South Melbourne, Victoria 3205, Australia

Chapman & Hall India, R. Seshadri, 32 Second Main Road, CIT East, Madras 600 035, India

First edition 1995

Typeset in 10/12 pt Ehrhardt by Best-set Typesetter Ltd., Hong Kong
Printed in Great Britain by St Edmundsbury Press, Bury St Edmunds, Suffolk

ISBN 0 412 56990 6

A catalogue record for this book is available from the British Library

Library of Congress Catalog Card Number: 94-72656

∞ Printed on permanent acid-free text paper, manufactured in accordance with ANSI/NISO Z39.48-1992 and ANSI/NISO Z39.48-1984 (Permanence of Paper).

Contents

Contributors

Professor H.S. Cronje
Obstetrics and Gynecology, University of the Orange Free State

Professor A. Tiltman
Anatomical Pathology, University of Cape Town

Dr G.M. Learmonth
Cytopathology Laboratory, University of Cape Town

Dr C.M. Durcan
Cytology Laboratory, University of Cape Town

J. Whittaker
Cytology Laboratory, University of Cape Town

Sister P. Stevens
Stomatherapy, Groote Schuur Hospital

Professor B. Lindeque
Obstetrics and Gynecology, University of Pretoria

Professor J. Knobel
Obstetrics and Gynecology, University of Pretoria

Professor B. Bloch
Gynecological Oncology, University of Cape Town

Dr C.M.C. Dehaeck
Gynecological Oncology, University of Cape Town

Dr R.P. Soeters
Gynecological Oncology, University of Cape Town

Professor E.W.W. Sonnendecker
Obstetrics and Gynecology, Witwatersrand University

Dr J. Nevin
Gynecological Oncology, University of Cape Town

Professor C. Falkson and G. Falkson
Medical Oncology, University of Pretoria

Dr L. van Wijk
Radiotherapy, University of Cape Town

Dr L. Denny
Gynecological Oncology, University of Cape Town

Dr H. Zungu
Traditional Healer, Kwa-Zuma, Johannesburg

Dr E. Sapire
Family Planning, University of Cape Town

Mrs L. Greef
Cancer Association of South Africa

Foreword

The authors have compiled a book of principles and guidelines which will be useful for students, practitioners and associated workers who may be responsible for large numbers of patients when only the essential facilities are available. Fortunately, good oncologic practice is possible even when the conditions are not ideal if the physicians train well in the characteristics of the disease. Various conditions in social and ethnic populations influence risk factors for genital tract cancers. Consideration of these factors is an important component in the design of cancer detection programs to achieve the greatest efficiency and dependability.

The results of treatment can be maximized if surgery, irradiation therapy and chemotherapy are equally available when selecting treatment. However, facilities for ultraradical operations, highly advanced technology for irradiation and the latest versions of chemotherapy contribute few additional cures over the more conventional and often more conservative treatments. The authors have provided the proper perspective for the role of more aggressive treatments. Their assessment may be reassuring to those who cannot offer this type of treatment to patients with advanced cancer or to those who have failed other treatments. When the number of patients exceeds the capacity of facilities and/or staff, the director must conserve energies and resources for patients who may benefit from treatment.

Everyone understands that advanced medical technology is beyond the reach of most Third World communities; it is beyond the need of most patients in industrialized nations, even though medical literature often heralds new technology as if it were essential. Technology has made significant contributions and hopefully those of proven value will be universally available. For the present we have not taken full advantage of our ability to discover early stage cancers for which treatment is more direct, simpler and curative. One needs only to look back in medical history and realize that the cure rates for various gynecologic cancers have made little gain due to our extravagant machines for imaging and complex laboratory tests for tumor products. Clearly they are helpful in monitoring the development and growth of cancers but used alone are not reliable for diagnosis.

Because there is a high incidence of cancer of the cervix and vulva in many countries with a dense population, screening programs and early detection efforts are very successful in finding cancers of the lower genital tract. Often these lesions are small and suited to local treatment. Physician directors of this work may have associated nurses or technicians who perform examinations and obtain the cytologic smears. These assistants can be taught colposcopy, obtain biopsies and, with physician decision and guidance, perform cryo or 'leep' therapy. This book has a chapter devoted to preinvasive lesions of the cervix, vagina and vulva. This material is essential in the care of large underprivileged populations who have high risk factors for genital tract squamous cancers. Two chapters discuss cytology and are very useful in training personnel for early detection programs.

The last four chapters concern the emotional consequences of cancer and its treatment. These are topics often omitted from our textbooks, yet are vital to the supportive care of the patient. Consequences of the disease and/or its treatment can pose many problems for the patient, whether these are real or imagined. It is essential that members of staff are able to counsel and reassure the patient. The chapter on psychosexual problems is well provided by its author.

Professor Bloch was a visiting professor at our institution when I first became acquainted with him. I appreciate his professional accomplishments. The editors are highly qualified to assemble this multiauthored treatise. Each has had extensive experience treating cancer patients. Their professional careers of teaching and research in academic institutions have prepared them for the selection of contributors with authoritative credentials. They have assembled within this volume knowledge that is current, yet the book is compact, economical and very readable. Duplications and conflicting recommendations among multiple contributors have been avoided.

I congratulate the editors and the contributors for their successful assembly of this information in a concise volume that is very readable and efficiently organized. The book will serve students well and be an excellent reference volume on the desk of the practitioner.

Felix N. Rutledge, M.D.
Professor of Gynecologic Oncology
University of Texas M.D. Anderson Cancer Centre

Preface

Working for many years in a country with both First and Third World patient components and problems in gynecological oncology we have become aware of many differences in disease patterns and presentation and in particular in the facilities available for the management of patients. With this background, when Katrien Dehaeck suggested that a manual for the many gynecological oncologists practising in under-developed countries would be of value we accepted the challenge. We are well aware that many excellent gynecological oncology textbooks are available and thus our aim is not to publish another comprehensive text. Rather we aim to satisfy the need for an affordable and easy reference guide to the management of patients with gynecological cancer in a setting where sophisticated and 'high tech' equipment is not available but where effective treatment is possible. Mention is made in the text of the value of such diagnostic and therapeutic methods but no detail is included.

We would like to thank our colleagues from other academic centers in our country for their contributions which were so willingly and timeously made. Without their co-operation it would not have been possible to complete this task.

Glaxo Pharmaceutical and their Medical Director, Dr Peter Moore, have supported this venture from the start and we are most grateful for all their assistance.

The manuscript was typed by Ms Nicole Ihle who had the unenviable task of interpreting illegible handwriting and unintelligible 'floppies'. We are most grateful to her for the dedication and the proficiency with which this task was performed.

It is our hope that this manual will be of value to our colleagues in Africa, South America, Asia and the rest of the developing world.

Basil Bloch
Katrien Dehaeck
Robbert Soeters
Gynecological Oncology Unit
Department of Obstetrics and Gynecology
University of Cape Town and Groote Schuur Hospital
Cape Town, South Africa

Editors' note: The provision of a gynecological oncology service

Our service which has operated for the past 30 years has been firmly based on the principle that the patient's best interests are served by a multidisciplinary team approach.

All new patients are seen initially at a Combined Assessment Clinic (CAC) after a routine clinical examination and metastatic screen. The members of the CAC are a radiotherapist with a special interest in gynecological cancer, a minimum of two gynecological oncologists and trainees, as well as two oncology trained sisters and support staff. A social worker is immediately available if required as are all auxiliary diagnostic methods and opinions from other disciplines. The individual patient is interviewed, examined by two members of the team and staging of the disease is determined. Thereafter management options are explained and a decision made regarding optimum treatment. An attempt is made to answer all the patient's questions, often through an interpreter, and arrangements are made to commence treatment as soon as possible.

The decision regarding treatment, whether surgical, radio- or chemotherapeutic is fully discussed, established protocols (reviewed regularly) are consulted and consensus opinion implemented. Surgery and chemotherapy are coordinated in the gynecological oncology unit (GOU) and radiotherapy in that department.

Follow-up clinics are held twice weekly, with special clinics for patients with ovarian cancer and trophoblastic disease.

Facilities are available for up-country patients to stay in residences provided by the Cancer Association of South Africa and good relationships are maintained with this organization and the Hospice movement to provide home and terminal care. A special effort is made to keep referring doctors and clinics informed regarding their patients' progress and to involve them in follow-up care.

We have found this to be an efficient, patient friendly system and would recommend it in countries such as ours.

1

Epidemiology of gynecological malignancies

H.S. Cronje

Epidemiology deals with the causes and distribution (including incidence) of disease. The causes of gynecological cancers are not known but significant data have been generated about the risk factors for developing a specific type of cancer, which will be addressed in this chapter.

VULVAR CANCER

Incidence

Cancer of the vulva is rare; it comprises only 3–5% of all **gynecological** cancers and only 1–2 per 100 000 women per year will develop the disease.

Risk factors for tumor development

It is thought that environmental factors play a major role but, presently, risk factors similar to those for cervical cancer are recognized. Important preceding or associated risk factors are leukoplakia of the vulva, inflammatory conditions of the vulva and vagina and urogenital cancer (mainly cervical cancer which is associated with vulvar carcinoma in 30% of cases). Vulvar intraepithelial neoplasia (VIN) has previously been regarded as a precursor of vulvar carcinoma. However, a small proportion (5% or less) of these will develop into cancer. The mean age for VIN is 25–30 years and for vulvar cancer 62–63 years.

Other risk factors identified for vulvar cancer are similar to those of cervical cancer. These include the following (with relative risks in brackets):

- Five or more lifetime sexual partners (RR 2.8)
- Age at first intercourse less than 18 years (RR 1.4)
- History of genital warts (RR 15.2)
- Previous abnormal Papanicolaou smear (RR 1.8)
- Current smoking (RR 2.0)
- History of sexually transmitted disease (RR 1.6). This was related mainly to genital warts and herpes
- Low socioeconomic status.

VAGINAL CANCER

Primary squamous cell carcinoma

Squamous cell carcinoma of the vagina is rare (1.8–2% of genital cancers) and occurs more often in older Black women of low educational and socioeconomic status. Morphologically it is similar to squamous carcinoma of the cervix. The only known risk factor is a history of genital warts. The well-known sexual risk factors for cervical cancer (early first sexual intercourse and multiple sexual partners) are not related to vaginal cancer and in a recent case-control study the following risk factors for vaginal cancer were identified:

- Vaginal discharge or irritation (RR 6.1)
- A previous abnormal Papanicolaou smear (RR 3.8)
- Previous hysterectomy, especially if done before the age of 40 years (RR 6.7)
- Vaginal trauma, including douching with preparations other than water or vinegar (RR 2.7)
- Frequent washing of the genital area (RR 2.7).

Adenocarcinoma of the vagina

In 1972 Herbst *et al.* reported eight cases of clear cell carcinoma of the vagina, thought previously very rare. Epidemiological studies demonstrated an association with maternal ingestion of diethylstilbestrol (DES) during the first trimester of pregnancy. The peak age frequency is 19.5 years and the risk of development of clear cell adenocarcinoma in a DES-exposed female until the age of 24 years is 0.14–1.4 per 1000.

Rare tumors

Sarcomas including sarcoma botryoides in children are rare. Other rare vaginal tumors are endodermal sinus tumors (also called mesonephroma or mesonephric carcinoma) and malignant melanoma.

CERVICAL CANCER

Cervical cancer has reached epidemic proportions in developing countries, including South Africa. The majority of cervical cancers are squamous cell carcinomas (about 95%), while a small (but increasing) proportion are adenocarcinomas.

Incidence

Cervical cancer is the most common cancer in women of low socio-economic status with the highest mortality rate. In developed societies, however, it is only the sixth most common malignancy in women. Countries with a high incidence include Colombia and Brazil, intermediate incidences are found in countries such as Germany, USA, India and Singapore, while low incidences were reported from Israel, UK, USA (Whites) and Sweden.

In South Africa cancer of the cervix is the most common malignancy in Black and Coloured women, second to breast cancer in Asian females and the fifth most common form of cancer in White women (Table 1.1). According to the Cancer Registry of South Africa there were 2897 cases of cervical cancer in South Africa in 1986, 2470 cases

Table 1.1 Most common malignancies in females in South Africa

White	Black
Basal Cell	Cervix
Breast	Breast
Colon	Esophagus
Melanoma	Uterus
Cervix	Mouth, Lip, Tongue, Pharynx, Liver
Coloured	**Asian**
Cervix	Breast
Breast	Cervix
Stomach	Uterus
Basal Cell	Stomach
Uterus	Rectum
Esophagus	Esophagus

Source: S. Africa Cancer Registry 1986 (corrected for age)

of basal cell carcinoma of the skin and 2350 cases of breast carcinoma, the three most common cancers in women. In Fig. 1.1 the age distribution for cervical cancer in South Africa is shown. The vast majority of these cancers were squamous cell carcinomas.

Several studies have been conducted in Southern Africa showing a high incidence of preinvasive lesions and cervical cancer. In a cytological screening program on 754 randomly chosen women in northern Namibia in 1988, a prevalence of 7.7% for cervical intraepithelial neoplasia (CIN) and 24.0% for human papilloma virus (HPV) infection was found. In Groote Schuur Hospital, Cape Town, the peak incidence for CIN is at 29–39 years and for invasive cancer 10 years later. The incidence of CIN in this hospital has shown a dramatic rise from 2.2 per 1000 smears in 1979 to 4.6 per 1000 in 1988. During the same period, HPV increased from 1.4 to 32.5 per 1000 smears. In Tygerberg Hospital, Cape Town, the rate of positive smears for CIN and invasive cancer was 9.3 per 1000 in 1978 and in the Transvaal an incidence of 10–31 per 100 000 for invasive cancer has been reported. A screening program in Soweto, Johannesburg, yielded detection rates, unequalled in the world literature, of 28 per 1000 for CIN and 13 per 1000 for invasive carcinomas. In Bloemfontein, cervical cancer accounts for 56% of all malignancies in Black women but only for 5% in White women.

Effect of cytological screening

Organized screening programs have a major impact on the reduction in mortality from cervical cancer. A prime example exists in the Nordic countries where mortality from cervical cancer was decreased by from 10% to 80%, depending on the efficiency of the program organization.

SQUAMOUS CELL CERVICAL CARCINOMA

This cancer is unique in several ways. It is situated on the surface of the cervix and therefore easily accessible, the precursors are well-known and cytology is a proven screening method.

Risk factors for tumor development

1. Coitus. Squamous cell carcinoma of the cervix appears to be a sexually transmitted disease due to its strong association with coitus and in particular multiple sexual partners; virgins almost never develop this form of cancer.

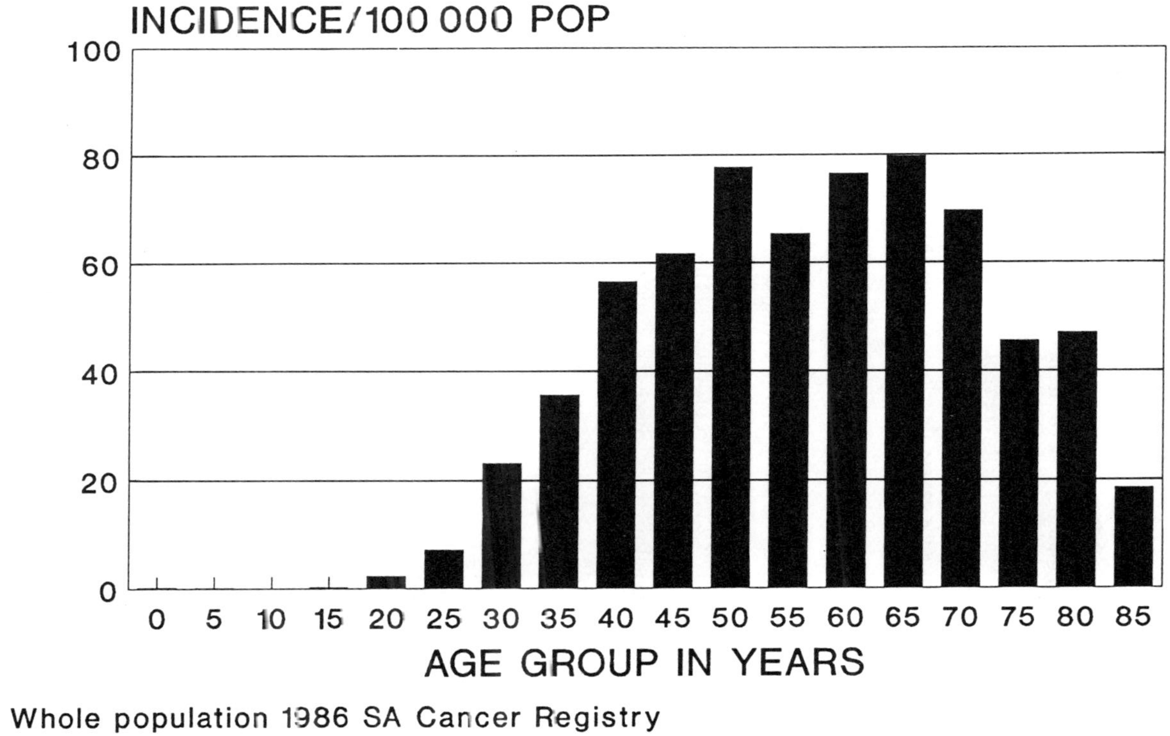

Fig. 1.1 Incidence of cervical cancer.

2. Socioeconomic factors. Cervical cancer is predominantly a disease of women in lower social classes, with the risk in the lowest social classes being about five times that among those in the highest classes.
3. Age of first intercourse. The younger a woman is at first intercourse, the higher her risk for developing cervical cancer. During and shortly after the menarche, marked ectopy exists. Soon these exposed endocervical cells are replaced by metaplastic squamous cells which if exposed to carcinogens become dysplastic (CIN) and eventually invasive cancer develops. Coitus is probably the vector of these carcinogens and the earlier the age of first intercourse, the more immature are the metaplastic cells and the more likely they are to become premalignant. In a virgin or when age at first intercourse was 19 years or more, the relative risk for developing cervical cancer is 1.00. If age at first intercourse were 17–18 years, the relative risk rises to 2.16. For 15–16 years it is 2.91 and for 15 years and younger it is 2.08 (lower probably due to small numbers in the reported studies).
4. Multiple sexual partners. Since the carcinogen(s) are likely to be transmitted sexually, the risk for cervical cancer will rise with an increase in the number of sexual partners. If the relative risk for cervical cancer is 1.00 for having none or one partner (now and in the past), it rises to 2.28 for two to four partners, 3.17 for five to nine partners and 3.27 for 10 or more partners.
5. The male factor: 'the high risk male'. The influence of the male partner has been demonstrated by geographic population clusters with high rates for both cervical and penile cancers. In addition, the wives of men with penile cancer have significantly elevated rates of cervical cancer. The most direct evidence for a male factor was from case-control studies where husbands of patients with cervical cancer had significantly more sexual partners than husbands of normal women.
6. Circumcision. Jewish women are known to have a low incidence of cervical cancer. This was attributed to the common practice of circumcision in Jewish males. Smegma, present in uncircumcised men, was considered a possible carcinogen but recent research has shown that this is not so. However, uncircumcized male partners remain an independant weak risk factor. Poor genital hygiene may be responsible for the effect.
7. Herpes simplex virus type 2 (HSV-2). In the 1970s several case-control studies showed significantly higher antibody levels to

HSV-2 in patients with cervical cancer compared with controls. Prospective studies, however, have been unable to demonstrate similar strong associations and a more recent prospective cohort study revealed no relationship between HSV-2 and subsequent cervical cancer.

8. Human papilloma virus (HPV). Recent investigations have focused on the possible role of HPV in the pathogenesis of cervical cancer. HPV types 6 and 11 are closely related to the development of condylomata acuminata and CIN 1 and types 16, 18 and 31 (and others to a lesser extent) to CIN 2 and 3 and cervical cancer. HPV types 6 and 11 are episomal and are not integrated into the host cell genome. On the other hand, HPV types 16 and 18 are, with rare exception, integrated into the viral DNA of the host. The mechanism of this transcription suggests that the virus has a role in the pathogenesis of this disease process.

   Women with CIN 3 associated with HPV infections are often 10 years younger than those with similar CIN but without HPV. Both in the USA and the UK a marked increase in the incidence of CIN was noted during the past 15 years with a high rate of progression to invasion. Australian women with HPV on their Papanicolaou smears, but without CIN, were followed prospectively and during the 6 years of follow-up these women had a 15 fold increase in the development of CIN 3 compared with that expected in the general population.

   Sexual consorts of patients with CIN have been evaluated for HPV infections and 90% have been identified as being positive and there is an established high risk of sexual transmission to their consorts (76%).

   The vector for carrying HPV from one person to another is a squamous epithelial cell. Although genital HPV is sexually transmitted in the majority of cases, other forms of transmission are rarely possible. It is important not to label this as a veneral disease when consulting with a patient. Stable marriages have been seriously traumatized by suggesting extramarital partners.

   HPV has thus been closely related to the pathogenesis of cervical cancer but some doubts have been expressed recently. Future studies will clarify this association.

9. Other infective agents. Many infective diseases, including syphilis and the common causes of vaginitis and endocervicitis, have been studied with respect to their possible role in carcinogenesis. None have been proved to be causally associated with the development

of cervical cancer. However, non-specific genital infection has a relative risk of 1.94 for developing cervical cancer.

10. Smoking. Smoking is regarded as a significant independent risk factor for squamous cell cancer with a relative risk for cancer development of 1.5. Long-term smokers, high-intensity smokers, and the use of non-filter cigarettes may increase the risk.
11. Alcohol. Alcohol is not a risk factor.
12. Race. The Black races have a higher rate of cervical cancer. This may be attributed to low socioeconomic status and other confounding variables. The evidence is not conclusive and a final conclusion cannot be reached at present.
13. Sperm proteins. Sperm proteins and even sperm heads have been found in metaplastic cervical epithelial cells. Their role in the pathogenesis of cervical cancer is not clear.
14. Oral contraceptives. Patients using oral contraceptives have a relative risk of 1.5 for the development of cervical cancer which rises to approximately 2.0 among long-term users after control for confounding variables. The mechanism for this increased risk is unclear.
15. Other contraceptive methods. Depo-medroxyprogesterone acetate (DMPA) is not associated with an increased risk. Barrier methods protect against cervical cancer.
16. Occupational factors. Prostitutes have high incidences of CIN and cervical cancer, probably related to multiple sexual partners. Husbands whose occupations necessitate prolonged absences from home are 'high risk males' and their spouses are also at increased risk. Extramarital affairs may account for this increase in risk.
17. Immunosuppression. Immunosuppressed patients are at increased risk for CIN but this risk has not been established for invasive cancer.
18. Dietary habits. Vitamin A, carotene, folic acid and vitamin C are apparently protective factors.
19. Parity. The number of births has again been found to be a risk factor (relative risk of 2.3 for four or more births) after it had previously been discounted.
20. Interval since last Papanicolaou smear. The relative risk for developing cervical cancer increases to 1.9 if the interval since the last Papanicolaou smear is 3–4 years and to 3.7 for an interval of 5 or more years. Women who have never had a smear have a relative risk of 4.26.

ADENOCARCINOMA OF THE CERVIX

Incidence

The incidence of adenocarcinoma of the cervix (ACC) was previously quoted at about 5% but recent studies have consistently reported rates of about 10%. This has been a consistent trend in recent world literature.

Risk factors

1. Sexual habits. Risk increases with earlier age at first intercourse and increasing number of sexual partners. These findings suggest a potential role for sexually transmitted and particularly viral factors.
2. Parity. An association between parity and risk of ACC has been reported.
3. Oral contraceptives. Due to the low incidence of ACC, no consistent association has been demonstrated.
4. Medical history. Excessive body weight, hypertension and diabetes mellitus are considered risk factors. Similarity therefore exists between the risk factors for endometrial cancer and ACC.
5. Socioeconomic class. Inconsistent findings have been reported.

ENDOMETRIAL CANCER

Incidence

Endometrial cancer is the fifth leading cancer in women worldwide and in South Africa. In developed countries it is the most common gynecological cancer but in developing countries it is surpassed by cervical cancer.

There is a wide difference in the incidence which is high in developed countries and variable among different racial groups. Developing countries (and Japan) have incidence rates four to five times lower. The incidence in South Africa is not known but among White women in the Orange Free State, it is at least five times higher than in Black women, while in the USA the incidence in White women is twice that in Black women.

Since endometrial cancer is a disease of elderly women, the incidence will increase as the population ages. Furthermore, higher rates are generally found in urban populations. In South Africa a high rate of urbanization is occurring which may influence the incidence of endometrial cancer in the future.

Risk factors for the development of endometrial cancer

1. Socioeconomic status. Higher socioeconomic status is related to a higher incidence of endometrial cancer but this association may have been influenced by hormonal replacement therapy and obesity which are both more common in women of higher socioeconomic class.
2. Body weight and height. With hormone replacement therapy (HRT), obesity is the most important risk factor for endometrial cancer and the latter relationship is stronger in women who have never used HRT.
3. Menstrual factors. The risk for endometrial cancer in women with a late menarche is about 50% less than those with an early menarche. Amenorrhea or irregular long menstrual cycles are associated with anovulation and unopposed estrogen stimulation and hence with an increased risk of endometrial cancer. A late menopause is associated with a 1.0–2.5 times greater risk.
4. Pregnancy and fertility. Nulliparous women have been consistently found to be at increased risk of endometrial cancer. A decrease in risk with increasing number of children has also been reported but less consistently. Infertility and polycystic ovarian syndrome rather than nulliparity could be related to the increased risk.
5. Estrogen replacement therapy. Since the early 1970s an association between unopposed estrogen use and endometrial cancer has been consistently demonstrated. The overall evidence suggests that the risk is about three to four times higher in 'ever' than 'never' users. This rises with duration of use and dose, there being a more than 10-fold elevation in women who had used high dose estrogens for 10 years or more.

   The addition of progestogens to estrogens in adequate dose (for at least 10 days of each treatment cycle) has been shown to protect against endometrial hyperplasia, considered an endometrial cancer precursor.
6. Anti-estrogens. Anti-estrogens (particularly Tamoxifen) may be associated with a twofold increase in endometrial cancer risk.
7. Oral contraceptive use. There is consistent evidence that combined oral contraceptives reduce the risk of endometrial cancer by about 50%.

8. Dietary factors. Positive correlations have been demonstrated between meat, eggs, milk, fats and oils, total proteins, fats and calorie intake and the incidence of the disease in developed countries. However, obesity and a lack of exercise may be confounding variables. Green vegetables and fresh fruit may have a protective effect.
9. Medical history. A history of diabetes mellitus and/or hypertension has been associated with an increased risk of endometrial cancer. Other associated diseases are arthritis and thyroid disease.
10. Smoking. Smoking has a protective effect, possibly because of the anti-estrogenic effect mediated by the induction of hepatic microsomal enzymes. Smokers have an early menopause, a higher incidence of osteoporosis and they tend to be leaner than non-smokers.
11. Family history. A positive family history is associated with a higher incidence of associated breast, ovarian and, to a lesser extent, colon carcinoma with an associated worse prognosis.

OVARIAN CANCER

Incidence

Epithelial ovarian cancer occurs most commonly in developed, industrialized countries with the exception of Japan. The three countries with the highest reported incidences are Sweden, Denmark and Switzerland, with cumulative incidences of 2.12, 2.03 and 1.91%. Countries with the lowest reported incidences are Senegal (0.38%), Japan (0.43%), China, Shanghai (0.47%) and Dutch Antilles (0.55%).

Ovarian cancer is the most common cause of death from gynecological cancer in the USA (52%) and the most common cancer to occur in advanced stage (67%). It is the sixth most common female cancer and the fourth most common cause of female cancer death.

Little is known about epidemiological characteristics of ovarian cancer in South Africa. In the USA, where 75–80% of ovarian tumors are of epithelial origin, 10% are stromal and 5% germ cell in origin but in the Western Cape area of South Africa 45% are epithelial, 11% stromal and 44% germ cell in origin. The increased prevalence of germ cell tumors (mainly benign cystic teratoma) was predominantly seen in Coloured and Black patients but not in Whites and Indians.

Etiology

The etiology of ovarian cancer is unknown but several risk factors have been identified.

1. Hereditary factors. A subset of ovarian cancer cases is now considered to have a genetic link. In the recently established Roswell Park Cancer Centre Familial Ovarian Cancer Registry 1336 cases in 587 families had been registered by the end of 1990.

   The most important risk factor is a first-degree relative with ovarian carcinoma from a familial ovarian cancer family. Such an individual has a 50% chance of developing the disease compared to 1.4% (1 in 70) with no family history. The inheritance factor is believed to be autosomal dominant and is possibly transmitted by males.

   The specific genetic abnormality that causes ovarian cancer has not been identified. Factors that have been implicated include the activation of proto-oncogenes and low levels of serum alpha-L-fucosidase. In addition, alterations in chromosomes 1, 3, 6 and 11 have frequently been associated with ovarian cancer.

   Inherited cancers frequently occur 10–15 years earlier than non-inherited cancers. In the above mentioned Registry, the mean age of the mothers was 60.3 years and the mean age of the daughters was 47.5 years ($p < 0.001$). The mean age of 23 266 women with ovarian cancer in the SEER data was 59.9 years.
2. Reproductive and endocrine factors.
   (a) Oral contraceptives
   Several studies have indicated that pregnancy and the use of oral contraceptives are protective against the development of ovarian cancer. The Centers for Disease Control reported that the use of oral contraceptives reduced the risk of ovarian cancer by 40% for women 20–54 years of age. This protective effect lasted for at least 10 years after oral contraceptive use was discontinued.
   (b) Pregnancy
   Similarly, the protective effect of pregnancy is in the order of 40% for women who have had two children. Thus, in addition to a positive family history, the absence of the use of oral contraceptives and nulliparity are two of the most identifiable risk factors for ovarian cancer.
   (c) Viral and blood group factors
   No convincing evidence exists of an association between viral infections (including mumps and rubella) and an increased

risk for ovarian cancer. Although an association has been suggested with blood group A the evidence is unconvincing.

3. Environmental and dietary factors. Epithelial ovarian cancer is related to affluent industrialized countries with the exception of Japan. However, first and second generations of Japanese women born in the USA have incidence rates approaching White women born in the USA.

   Because of the association between an industrialized environment and epithelial ovarian cancer, a large number of possible etiological factors have been investigated, of which asbestos, talc and diet are the most important.

   (a) Asbestos and talc. Asbestos is a known carcinogen causing malignant mesothelioma. Talc (hydrous magnesium silicate) in powder form often contained asbestos until recently. Conceptually, talcum powder on the perineum could reach the ovaries by passage through the vagina or cervix.
   (b) Diet. A high intake of meat and animal fat and a high consumption of yoghurt, cottage cheese and whole milk have been associated with a high incidence of ovarian cancer. No association has been found between ovarian cancer and the use of coffee, alcohol or tobacco.

4. Experimental tumorgenesis. The experimental induction of ovarian tumors in animals usually produces stromal tumors. Methods used include the use of carcinogens (e.g. 7,12-dimethylbenz anthracene or DMBA), X-rays, gonodotropins and transplants.

2

Pathology of gynecological neoplasms

A. Tiltman

PATHOLOGY

This chapter discusses the macroscopic and microscopic morphology of selected gynecological tumors and those morphologic features which may indicate prognosis. Discussion of the epidemiology, etiology, pathogenesis, spread, stage and behavior will be found elsewhere.

VULVA

Tumors of the vulva may arise from the skin and mucosa, urethra, the adnexal glands, ectopic breast tissue and soft tissue as well as a miscellaneous group including lymphomas and neuroectodermal tumors.

The most common are those of epithelial origin.

- Squamous carcinoma
- Basal cell carcinoma
- Melanoma
- Paget's disease.

Squamous carcinoma

The precursor lesions of squamous carcinoma of the vulva (vulval intraepithelial neoplasia or VIN I, II, III) and the part played by human papillomavirus in the genesis of carcinoma are discussed elsewhere (Chapter 1).

Squamous carcinoma may arise anywhere on the skin or mucosa of the vulva. Multifocal carcinomas may occur in up to 30% of cases. Microscopically, keratin is present in most instances and may be excessive. Invasion of the underlying tissues may take place in a tentacular (stellate) or pushing (broad front) fashion.

Verrucous carcinoma has a pronounced papillary (warty) structure and is a very well-differentiated squamous carcinoma microscopically. Diagnosis requires adequate deep biopsy.

MORPHOLOGIC INDICATORS OF PROGNOSIS

1. Size. Carcinomas greater than 2 cm in diameter have a fourfold greater risk of lymph node metastases than smaller tumors.
2. Grade. Approximately 90% of squamous carcinomas of the vulva are well or moderately differentiated (grades 1 and 2). These grades are not well-defined morphologically. They can be easily distinguished from grade 3 (poorly differentiated) but not so easily from each other. From 16 to 33% of grade 1, 28 to 48% of grade 2 and 62 to 75% of grade 3 tumors have lymph node metastases.
3. Depth of invasion. Increasing depth of invasion of vulval carcinoma is associated with a higher incidence of lymph node metastases and lower survival. However, several different methods to measure depth of invasion have been used so that direct comparison of results is difficult. The **depth of invasion** may be defined as the distance between the basement membrane at the top of the most superficial adjacent dermal papilla to the deepest point of invasion. When so defined, lymph node metastases are not found with tumors showing less than 1 mm stromal invasion. Tumors with more than 1 mm but less than 3 mm invasion have a 12% chance of lymph node metastases and when more than 5 mm a 15% chance.

   A technically easier and more reproducible measurement is **tumor thickness** measured from the surface to the deepest point of invasion. When the tumor thickness is less than 3 mm metastases have not been observed.
4. Vascular channel invasion. This is associated with a higher incidence of lymph node metastases. It is a better indicator in well and moderately differentiated carcinomas (vessel invasion absent/present = 16%/67%) than the poorly differentiated (60%/67%).

Basal cell carcinoma

This tumor of the vulva is uncommon, usually ulcerated and behaves in a locally aggressive fashion.

Melanomas

These tumors of the vulva are also uncommon. They are usually nodular in type and behave as melanomas elsewhere. Prognosis depends mostly on depth of invasion.

Paget's disease

This disease of the vulva is the presence of adenocarcinoma cells lying within the epidermis. It may be associated with an adenocarcinoma of an underlying adnexal gland and may also show stromal invasion.

VAGINA

The vast majority of neoplasms in the vagina are metastatic either as a result of direct extension from the cervix, vulva, bladder, urethra and rectum or as a result of lymphatic or blood spread from the endometrium or ovary.

The most common primary malignant tumors are:

- Squamous carcinoma
- Adenocarcinoma
- Sarcomas
- Melanoma.

Squamous carcinoma

Primary squamous carcinoma of the vagina is usually preceded by dysplasia and carcinoma *in situ* (vaginal intraepithelial neoplasia or VaIN I, II and III) but the single greatest risk factor is a previous carcinoma of the cervix or vulva. The macroscopic and microscopic morphology is similar to squamous carcinomas of the vulva. There are no reliable indicators of prognosis.

Adenocarcinoma

This is uncommon except in those individuals who have been exposed to DES *in utero* where they occur in the upper vagina in relation to vaginal adenosis. In older women clear cell carcinomas of the vagina occur rarely.

Sarcomas

Sarcomas of the vagina are rare and include:

- Rhabdomyosarcoma which occurs in young children and presents as a polypoid mass of pale or grey myxomatous tissue at the introitus (sarcoma botryoides)
- Leiomyosarcoma which occurs is older women and may present with a non-polypoid mass composed of smooth muscle.

Melanomas

These occur infrequently in the vagina and usually present as pigmented lesions on the mucosa.

UTERINE CERVIX

Carcinoma of the uterine cervix can be classified on histological grounds into five groups.

- Squamous carcinoma
- Adenocarcinoma
- Mixed adenosquamous carcinomas
- Undifferentiated carcinoma
- A miscellaneous group

With the exception of undifferentiated carcinomas each of these categories contains several morphologic subtypes.

Squamous carcinoma

The precursor to invasive squamous carcinoma is CIN. This lesion and the role of human papillomavirus in the genesis of cervical carcinoma are discussed in Chapters 1 and 2.

Squamous carcinomas arise in the transformation zone and are usually visible on the ectocervix (Fig. 2.1). Occasional squamous car

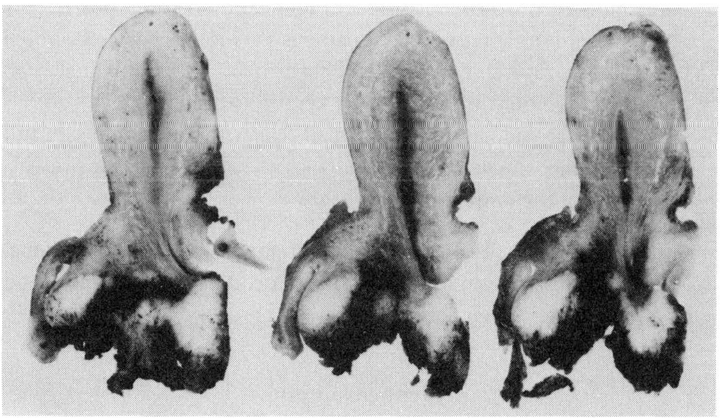

Fig. 2.1 Three parasagittal slices through a uterus. The anterior is on the right. The posterior lip of the cervix is replaced by an exophytic carcinoma protruding into the upper vagina.

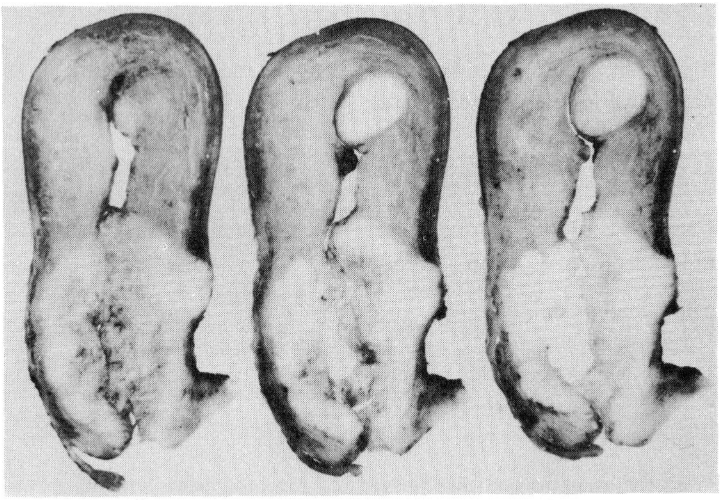

Fig. 2.2 Three parasagittal slices through a uterus showing a squamous carcinoma high in the endocervical canal producing a 'barrel-shaped cervix'. The ectocervix appears normal. The lesion in the fundus is a fibromyoma.

cinomas arise and grow within the endocervical canal producing the so called 'barrel-shaped cervix' and are not readily visible on vaginal or colposcopic examination (Fig. 2.2).

Microscopically three cell types are described:

1. Large cell, keratinizing squamous carcinoma composed of typical squamous cells with whorls of cells and central keratin pearls.
2. Large cell, non-keratinizing squamous carcinoma has cells which are recognizably squamous. There may be individual cell keratinization but no extracellular keratin is present.
3. Small cell carcinomas consist of small cells with little cytoplasm and darkly stained nuclei. Occasional foci of keratin may be present, establishing their squamous heritage.

Verrucous carcinoma is an uncommon variant of squamous carcinoma. Correct diagnosis depends on an adequate deep biopsy and good clinicopathologic correlation.

Adenocarcinoma

Adenocarcinomas arise from the cells of the endocervical crypts. The precursor lesions include adenocarcinoma *in situ* which is recognized by cellular atypia confined to the crypts. Microscopically, five cell types may be seen either in pure or mixed form.

1. Endocervical type is composed of columnar cells containing intracytoplasmic mucin.
2. Endometrioid type contains cells and glands resembling those seen in the endometrium. Mucin is not present.
3. Clear cell type is composed of cells with clear cytoplasm containing glycogen. These cells may be arranged in sheets or in acinar formations.
4. An intestinal type with goblet cells is an uncommon form.
5. Poorly differentiated adenocarcinomas present sheets of cells, the majority of which contain intracytoplasmic mucin.

Minimal deviation adenocarcinoma (adenoma malignum) is a rare, very well-differentiated carcinoma of endocervical type. Because of the extremely good differentiation of these tumors the correct, early diagnosis requires good clinicopathologic correlation.

Mixed adenosquamous carcinomas

These tumors contain both recognizable squamous and glandular elements. A mucin stain should be performed routinely on all cervical carcinomas to demonstrate the possible presence of glandular elements.

MORPHOLOGIC INDICATORS OF PROGNOSIS

1. Size. Increasing size of the primary tumor is associated with a poorer prognosis.
2. Cell type. Adenocarcinomas are generally regarded as having a poorer prognosis than squamous carcinomas but this is true only for tumors more advanced than stage I.

   Whether differences in cell type of squamous carcinomas have any bearing on prognosis is controversial and still requires elucidation.
3. Depth of invasion. There is a direct correlation between depth of invasion, lymph node metastases and survival.
4. Vascular channel invasion. This is generally regarded as being associated with a higher incidence of lymph node metastases and a poorer prognosis but is not always easy to identify with confidence.

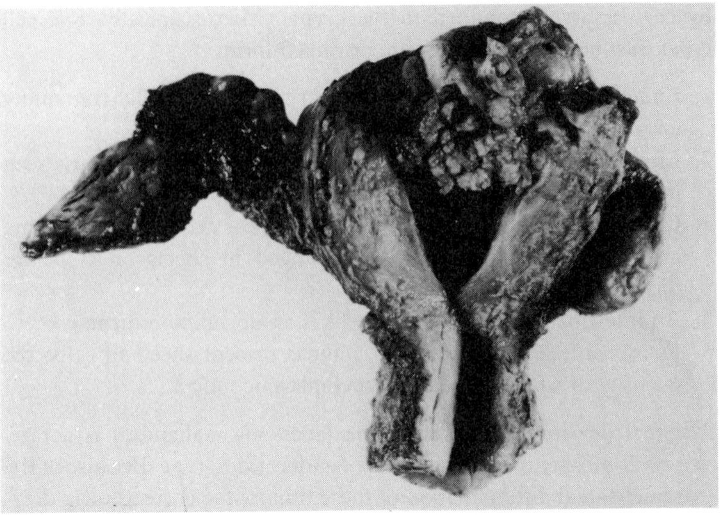

Fig. 2.3 Uterus opened anteriorly to show a polypoid carcinoma in the fundus.

ENDOMETRIUM

Tumors of the endometrium may be classified into:

- Epithelial: carcinoma
- Stromal: sarcoma
- Mixed epithelial stromal.

Endometrial carcinoma

Carcinomas may arise anywhere in the endometrial cavity but generally occur more frequently in the fundus often extending into the cornua (Fig. 2.3). Extension into the myometrium, when present, is usually visible to the naked eye and the depth of invasion and distance from the serosal surface is best measured during gross examination.

Microscopically varying cell types and architectures may be found in either mixed or pure form.

1. Endometrioid adenocarcinoma. This is the usual form of endometrial adenocarcinoma. Morphologic variants are:
   (a) With squamous differentiation. Adenocarcinoma with squamous metaplasia (adenoacanthoma) or adenosquamous carcinoma.
   (b) Secretory carcinoma shows cytoplasmic vacuolation.
   (c) Ciliated cell carcinoma.

2. High grade uterine papillary carcinoma (UPC). This is composed of pleomorphic cuboidal cells morphologically similar to those seen in serous carcinomas of the ovary and was originally described as uterine papillary serous carcinoma. An admixture of clear cell may be present. The architecture is usually distinctly papillary with well-developed fibrovascular cores covered by stratified tumor cells. In some areas there may be an acinar pattern. Psammoma bodies may be present. This tumor has a high propensity to invade deeply into the myometrium and to invade lymphatic vessels. There is often wide dissemination throughout the peritoneal cavity.
3. Clear cell adenocarcinoma is composed of cells with clear cytoplasm and large pleomorphic nuclei. The cytoplasm contains glycogen. The cells are arranged in sheets, acini or in papillary formations.
4. Mucinous adenocarcinoma is uncommon and composed predominantly of cells with intracytoplasmic mucin.
5. Squamous carcinoma is rare.
6. Undifferentiated carcinoma.

MORPHOLOGIC INDICATORS OF PROGNOSIS

1. Cell type.
   (a) Clear cell carcinomas have been reported as having a poorer prognosis than usual endometrial carcinoma (64% vs 80% 5 year survival).
   (b) Adenosquamous carcinomas have previously been regarded as being more aggressive than endometrioid carcinoma but the behavior of carcinomas with squamous metaplasia depends on the grade of the glandular element.
2. Papillary growth pattern. High grade uterine papillary carcinomas have a poorer prognosis (with five times the relapse rate) than the usual forms of endometrial carcinoma. This is related to the high nuclear grade of these tumors. Papillary neoplasms of endometrioid type have been shown to have an intermediate progression rate between UPC and endometrioid adenocarcinomas.
3. Grade. Endometrial carcinomas are graded according to architectural patterns:
   (a) Grade 1: 5% or less of the non-squamous element show solid growth.
   (b) Grade 2: 6–50% of non-squamous show solid growth.
   (c) Grade 3: more than 50% of non-squamous element show solid growth.

Significant nuclear atypia (high nuclear grade) raises the grade by one.

High grade tumors are associated with a higher frequency of lymph node metastases and a poorer prognosis.

4. Depth of myometrial invasion. More than 50% of myometrial thickness is related to a poorer prognosis.
5. Vascular channel invasion. This is an independent prognostic indicator for recurrence but is more frequently present in high grade tumors.

Endometrial stromal sarcoma

Three lesions may develop from the endometrial stroma.

1. Stromal nodule is a benign, usually small, discrete nodule in the endometrium.
2. Low grade stromal sarcoma is a tumor of low malignancy. Characteristically it extends into the myometrium in a finger-like fashion through vascular and lymphatic spaces (endolymphatic stromal myosis). Microscopically there are less than 10 mitoses/10 high power fields (10 HPF) and the nuclei are bland. [The use of 10 high power fields has become standard in the literature but the area of a microscopic high power field is not uniform between microscopes. Unit area is preferable, i.e. 1 mm^2 is approximately the same area as 10 HPF].
3. High grade stromal sarcoma microscopically shows some nuclear atypia and more than 10 mitoses/10 HPF. Invasion into the myometrium may be extensive.

Mixed epithelial stromal neoplasms

This group of neoplasms has given rise to considerable difficulties with nomenclature due largely to lack of understanding as to their pathogenesis.

Two malignant tumors in this group need description.

1. Adenosarcoma is an uncommon tumor composed of a malignant stroma with a benign epithelial component.
2. Carcinosarcoma (malignant mixed Müllerian tumor (MMMT); mixed mesodermal tumor; metaplastic carcinoma) is a tumor composed of malignant stromal and epithelial components (Fig. 2.4). The stromal elements may be homologous to those found in the uterus (endometrial stroma, fibrosarcoma, leiomyosarcoma) and/or

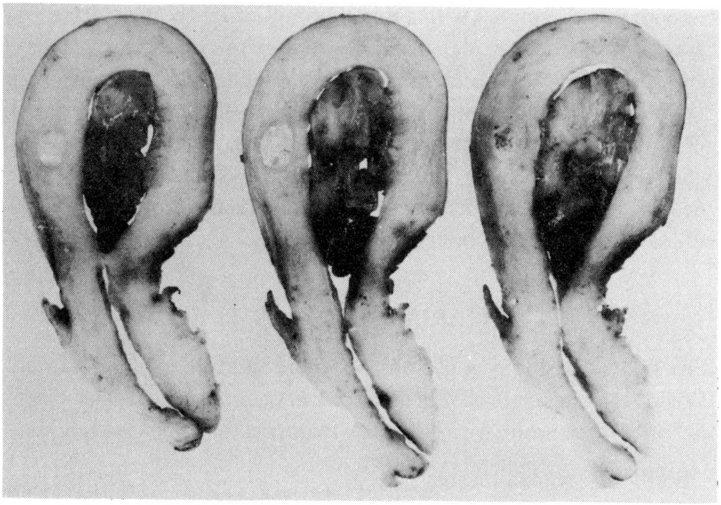

Fig. 2.4 Three parasagittal slices showing a malignant mixed Müllerian tumor filling the endometrial cavity and arising from a narrow stalk on the anterior wall.

heterologous (rhabdomyosarcoma, chondrosarcoma, osteosarcoma). The epithelial component may be any of those seen in endometrial carcinomas but is frequently undifferentiated.

Morphologic indicators of prognosis

1. Cell type. While there is some disagreement in the literature, the different sarcomatous elements have no relation to behavior. It is the grade or type of epithelial component that is related to prognosis.
2. Depth of invasion, stage and involvement of the lower uterine segment or endocervix are all associated with a poorer prognosis.

MYOMETRIUM

Leiomyosarcomas are usually softer in consistency than leiomyomas. They may contain areas of necrosis or hemorrhage. The borders may be irregular and show infiltration into the surrounding myometrium. Microscopically they usually show typical smooth muscle cells arranged in bundles. Cellular pleomorphism varies from minimal to marked. The diagnosis of malignancy is based on mitotic activity.

Smooth muscle tumors with a mitotic count of 10 mitoses/10 HPF or more are regarded as malignant. Tumors with counts of between 5 and 9/10 HPF should, in the absence of cellular pleomorphism, be regarded as of uncertain malignant potential but in the presence of pleomorphism should be regarded as a low grade sarcomas. These figures are guidelines only. Progestational agents, particularly medroxyprogesterone, may cause both increases in mitotic activity and cellular pleomorphism in benign leiomyomas.

OVARIAN NEOPLASMS

The WHO classification of ovarian tumors and tumor-like conditions contains 14 categories of which 12 refer to possible primary neoplasms and only three occur with sufficient frequency to be considered here:

- Epithelial-stromal tumors
- Sex cord/stromal tumors
- Germ cell tumors.

EPITHELIAL-STROMAL TUMORS

The epithelial-stromal tumors of the ovary are subclassified initially by cell type.

1. Serous tumors are composed of cells resembling the lining cells of the fallopian tube or the surface mesothelium of the ovary. Cilia may be present. Mucin may be produced but is demonstrable only at the cell surface. Psammoma bodies may be present.
2. Mucinous tumors are composed of cells with intracytoplasmic mucin. These cells may be tall columnar and resemble those seen in the endocervix or goblet cells resembling those of the intestinal mucosa. The latter may be associated with argyrophil cells.
3. Endometrioid tumors contain cells resembling those usually found in the endometrium. Squamous metaplasia may be present. Extra cellular mucin may be found. Mixed Müllerian tumors of the ovary are included in this category.
4. Clear cell tumors are composed of cells with a clear cytoplasm and pleomorphic nuclei. The cells contain abundant glycogen.
5. Transitional cell tumors show urothelial differentiation with nests of polygonal cells characteristically showing a nuclear groove.
6. Mixed epithelial tumors contain more than one cell type each in a significant amount.
7. Undifferentiated tumors.

Each of these tumor types (with the exception of undifferentiated carcinoma) can be subdivided according to malignant potential.

1. Benign tumors contain cells with no cytologic atypia or other features of malignancy and are not considered further.
2. Tumors of borderline malignancy (or carcinoma of low malignant potential) (Fig. 2.5) show some but not all the morphologic features of malignancy. By definition, no stromal invasion is present but because of the complex architectural structure of some of these tumors, particularly in mucinous borderline tumors, the presence or absence of stromal invasion may be difficult to identify. A sufficient number of blocks needs to be examined. The accepted norm would be one block per centimeter tumor diameter. Serous borderline tumors typically show a papillary architecture covered by stratified cells with tufting and apparent detachment of small clusters of cells. Some degree of cellular atypia is present but not marked. Recent reports have described serous borderline tumors with microinvasion which have shown the same good prognosis. Mucinous borderline tumors are more usually the intestinal type but Müllerian mucinous borderline tumors with endocervicoid cells

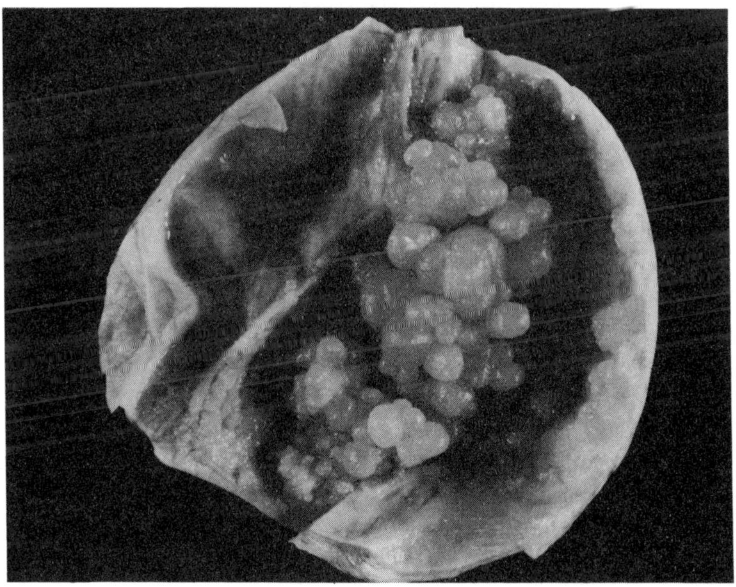

Fig. 2.5 Serous tumor of borderline malignancy with coarse and fine papillary structures on the inner surface of the cyst.

do occur. The tumor cells show nuclear atypia, mitotic activity and stratification. Stratification to more than four cell layers has been regarded as indicative of carcinoma.

Endometrioid, clear cell and transitional cell borderline tumors are uncommon and show cytological and architectural atypia between benign adenoma and carcinoma.

3. Malignant tumors show all the morphologic features of malignancy. Stromal invasion is usually present.

The frequency of bilateral primary epithelial tumors of the ovary is around 10%. Benign and borderline endometrioid, clear cell and transitional cell tumors are uncommon and statistics for bilaterality are not available. It is not clear why the figures for Cape Town are lower than the others. They are based on a relatively small number of cases but provisional results from a survey of over 900 epithelial tumors show a similar trend with low percentage bilaterality for all serous, mucinous and endometrioid tumors.

Morphologic indicators of prognosis

1. Cell type. Possibly endometrioid and mucinous carcinoma share a better prognosis than other cell types.
2. Histological grade is the best prognostic indicator but while there is significant difference between grade 1 and grade 3 tumors this is not true between grades 1 and 2.

SEX CORD/STROMAL TUMORS

These tumors are thought to arise from derivatives of the primitive sex cords and/or the specialized stroma of the ovarian cortex. They may be divided into two groups: granulosa-stromal tumors and Sertoli-stromal tumors.

Granulosa-stromal tumors

1. Two forms of granulosa cell tumors exist: an adult and a juvenile type.
   (a) The adult type granulosa cell tumor is more common. The solid portions of the tumor show a yellow or cream colored appearance.

   Microscopically, the polygonal cells contain uniform nuclei with a diffuse chromatin pattern. The nuclei may show a nuclear groove. Various patterns of growth are described. The microfollicular forms presents the classical appearance with so-called Call–Exner bodies. The macrofollicular pattern resembles more the developing follicle. Less differentiated patterns include the insular, trabecular or sarcomatoid forms.

(b) The juvenile granulosa cell tumor occurs in patients less than 30 years old and is the more common form of granulosa cell tumor seen before puberty.

Microscopically the tumor cells contain a moderate amount of cytoplasm which may be luteinized. The nuclei are frequently hyperchromatic and pleomorphic. Mitoses may be frequent.

2. Theco-fibromatous tumors are generally benign. Macroscopically they are firm solid tumors but may show some cystic degeneration. The cut surface shows a whorled appearance which is grey/white but may show yellow areas if luteinized. Fibrosarcomas are defined as fibrous tumors having more than three mitoses per 10 HPF and appear similar macroscopically.

Morphologic indicators of prognosis

There are few reliable morphologic indicators of prognosis in stage 1 granulosa cell tumors. Large tumor size and a large number of mitoses are related to a poorer prognosis. Despite the pleomorphism of the juvenile type the prognosis is better than the adult form.

Sertoli-stromal tumors

1. Sertoli stromal cell tumors with well-developed tubules, with or without Leydig cells, generally behave in a benign fashion.
2. Malignant Sertoli stromal tumors show varying microscopic appearances.

Morphologic indicators of prognosis

Poorly differentiated tumors are more malignant than those of intermediate differentiation and tumors with more than 15 mitoses/10 HPF have a poorer prognosis.

GERM CELL TUMORS

1. Mature cystic teratomas are the most common ovarian germ cell tumor and in Southern Africa the most common of all ovarian

tumors. They are usually single and unilateral and approximately 10% are bilateral. Macroscopically they present with a single cyst filled with sebaceous material. Somewhere in the wall there is a nodule often containing adipose tissue and surmounted by a tuft of hair. Cartilage, bone and teeth may be present. Occasional cysts are filled with clear straw-colored fluid.

Mature cystic teratomas are benign but about 1% may undergo malignant transformation and this is most frequently a squamous carcinoma. Carcinoids and adenocarcinoma are less common and other tumors such as melanoma and sarcomas have been described.

2. Immature teratomas are usually unilateral and are large at presentation. Macroscopically they show both solid and cystic areas but the cysts may be very small (Fig. 2.6). Microscopically they contain immature (fetal-like) tissues. Immature neuroectodermal tissues are often prominent. Interspersed between the immature elements are mature tissues. Immature teratomas are graded on the relative proportions of mature to immature constituents and it is important to

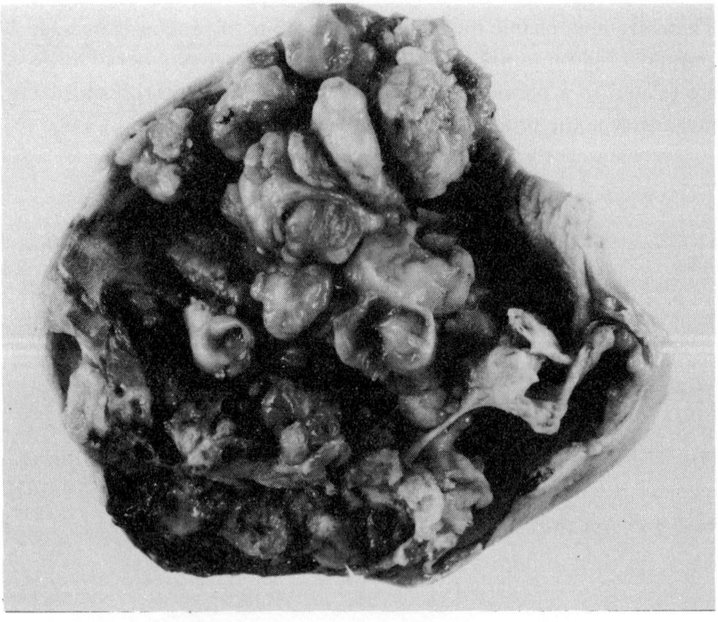

Fig. 2.6 Immature teratoma. The cut surface shows nodules of solid, white, neuroectodermal tissue within a larger cyst.

adequately sample the tumor. One block for each centimeter greatest diameter should be examined. While all immature tissues should be considered in grading it is the neuroectodermal component which dominates.

3. Dysgerminoma is a rare malignant tumor. It is bilateral in 5–10% of cases. Macroscopically they are usually solid with a soft or rubbery consistency. The surface is smooth but is often bosselated. The cut surface is cream colored. Microscopically there are sheets of uniform large polygonal cells. The cytoplasm may be clear and contain glycogen. Lymphocytes are usually present and there may be histiocytic giant cells.
4. Yolk sac tumors are uncommon. Microscopically the appearance resembles the extra embryonal yolk sac structures. Hyaline globules are typically present and alpha-feto protein and/or alpha-antitrypsin may be demonstrated in these.
5. Embryonal carcinoma is a rare malignant tumor which macroscopically often shows necrosis and hemorrhage and microscopically is composed of pleomorphic cuboidal cells often arranged in tubuloacinar structures.
6. Trophoblastic germ cell tumors or non-gestational choriocarcinoma have the same microscopic morphology as the gestational form. Both cyto- and syncytiotrophoblast may be present and beta HCG can be demonstrated.
7. Mixed germ cell tumors may occur containing mixtures of any of the above.

Morphologic indicators of prognosis

Cell Type. The presence of yolk sac, choriocarcinomatous or high grade immature teratomatous elements confers a poorer prognosis in both pure and mixed tumors. There are no other reliable morphologic indicators of prognosis.

If there is spread beyond the ovary the tumor is a borderline or frankly malignant tumor. If, however, it is confined to the ovary the distinction between benign and malignant may be difficult. If an intraoperative, frozen section, pathology opinion is available it should be requested.

In the absence of a frozen section service the macroscopic appearance of the tumors may be of help.

1. Cystic tumors with no papillary projections on either surface are usually benign.

2. Mucinous cystic tumors with a nodule composed of more solid tissue with smaller (micro) cysts should be regarded with great suspicion of malignancy.
3. Cystic or solid tumors with delicate surface papillary projections are most likely borderline or malignant tumors.
4. Solid tumors with small or tiny microcysts are more likely to be malignant.
5. Solid tumors with a firm consistency and no microcysts are more likely benign (fibrothecomas, Brenner tumors, adenofibromas etc.) except in young patients when they should be regarded with suspicion.

HYDATIDIFORM MOLE

1. Complete hydatidiform mole is typically diploid with all the genetic material being derived from the male. Macroscopically there is hydropic swelling of the majority of the chorionic villi. No fetus or fetal parts are present. Microscopically the villi are avascular and contain a central cistern presenting as a space filled with proteinaceous fluid only. Trophoblastic proliferation is always present but this varies from minimal and focal to marked and generalized. Proper sampling is required. The proliferating trophoblast contains both cyto- and syncytiotrophoblast and may show varying degrees of pleomorphism.
2. Partial hydatidiform mole is frequently triploid resulting from the fertilization of a normal ovum by two spermatozoa.

   Macroscopically there is hydropic swelling of only some of the villi and usually it is not as marked as seen in the complete mole. A fetus is usually present but as it usually dies early in pregnancy it may be difficult to find.

   Microscopically the swollen villi contain a central cistern. The villi may show a scalloped outline with trophoblast protruding into and sometimes included in the villus. Non-hydropic villi contain fetal blood vessels and may be fibrotic. Trophoblast proliferation is seldom marked and only focally hyperplastic.
3. Invasive hydatidiform mole is characterized by the presence of molar tissue invading the myometrium or at distant sites. Myometrial invasion should only be diagnosed in hysterectomy specimens and not curettings. While most invasive moles are complete, an invasive incomplete mole has been described.

   Microscopically the molar tissue is frequently seen within blood vessels. Trophoblastic proliferation is variable.

CHORIOCARCINOMA

Choriocarcinoma may follow any normal, ectopic or molar pregnancy and may occasionally be found in apparently normal placentae.

Macroscopically the tumor fills the endometrial cavity and invades the myometrium often extending into the broad ligament. It is generally hemorrhagic and necrotic.

Microscopically it is composed of both cyto- and syncytiotrophoblast which may show considerable pleomorphism. Except when occurring in a normal pregnancy, chorionic villi are absent. Invasion into vascular spaces is characteristic. Hemorrhagic necrosis is usually prominent.

PLACENTAL-SITE TROPHOBLASTIC TUMOR

Placental-site trophoblastic tumor (PSTT) (trophoblastic pseudotumor) is a tumor of extravillous trophoblast.

It may form a polypoid tumor protruding into the endometrial cavity but is largely a diffusely infiltrating lesion into the myometrium. Hemorrhage and necrosis is not a prominent feature. Microscopically the tumor cells are mainly mononuclear but some multinucleate cells are present. The cells invade as cords or individually between muscle fibers. Larger sheets of cells may be seen away from the invading edge. Non-destructive vascular invasion, similar to that seen in the normal placental site, is present but unlike choriocarcinoma, uninvolved vessels may be present within the tumor.

There are no reliable morphologic indicators of prognosis.

3

Cytology of the cervix: screening programs

G. Learmonth and C.M. Durcan

INTRODUCTION

Cancer of the uterine cervix is the most common cancer in women living in developing countries and is undoubtedly the only cancer that is potentially preventable. Early precancerous changes can be detected by cervical smears, taken with the Ayre spatula, and effectively treated. To achieve this a system of adequate follow-up must be established. The prerequisites for any screening program are:

1. Well-motivated, well-educated nursing or medical staff, to ensure good representative smears.
2. Highly trained cytotechnologists to ensure accurate screening.
3. Adequate laboratory facilities to ensure proper technical preparations of slides and good microscopes to reduce eyestrain.
4. A well trained cytopathologist.
5. A medical officer in charge of laboratory procedures to ensure proper supervision of screening and tracing and to liaise with gynecologists and to compile annual reports.
6. One or two tracing clerks to trace defaulters.
7. Effective population education and recruitment on a national basis.

The latter task is of the utmost importance in a Third World situation as poverty, unemployment, teenage pregnancies, cultural differences and overcrowding in shanty towns lead to an unstable, mobile population. Furthermore, women change their names frequently (when they marry, move to an urban area, change jobs etc.) making tracing notoriously difficult.

A population screening program for many developing countries including South Africa has not been established. At present 'opportunistic' screening is done at antenatal clinics, day hospitals, family planning clinics and hospital outpatient departments.

Taking the particular circumstances in the Republic of South Africa and other developing countries into account, the following is suggested as a suitable cost-effective program which would identify the vast majority of precancerous lesions. The screening intervals are practical and satisfy the above requirements.

1. The first cervical smear is to be taken as soon as possible (at first presentation) after the commencement of sexual activity, whatever age that might be.
2. Subsequent smears are to be taken at age 20 years and at 5 yearly intervals thereafter to age 70 years.

OR

3. Every sexually active woman to have at least three free cytologic smears during her lifetime at ages 25, 35 and 45 years. Additional smears to be arranged and paid for individually.
4. Repeat smears thereafter as follows:
   (a) With a minor abnormality (atypia to CIN 1) repeat in 1 year.
   (b) After minor abnormalities in three successive smears – refer for colposcopy.
   (c) Smears with CIN 2 and 3 – refer for colposcopy.
5. Follow-up smears for patients who have been treated for any abnormality to be taken every 6 months for 3 years and annually thereafter.

TAKING AN ADEQUATE CERVICAL SMEAR

The aim for every smear take is that it should be adequate, i.e. contain both endocervical and ectocervical cells which are evaluable. Adequate facilities are essential and include appropriately sized vaginal speculae, light, spatulae (Ayres), glass slides and fixative. The person taking the smear should be well trained and should be able to locate and identify the cervix.

The patient should be informed and reassured, comfortable and relaxed and the entire cervix visualized (Fig. 3.1). Cell samples should be taken from the ecto and endocervix and the entire transformation zone smeared onto a labeled glass slide and immediately fixed. Smears are most frequently classed as 'inadequate' due to an absence of endocervical cells and when in doubt a separate sample from the endocervix should be taken with a cytobrush or other appropriate sampler. The latter may be particularly necessary in post-menopausal women or patients on Depo Provera.

Cervical smears are best taken at mid-menstrual cycle when the

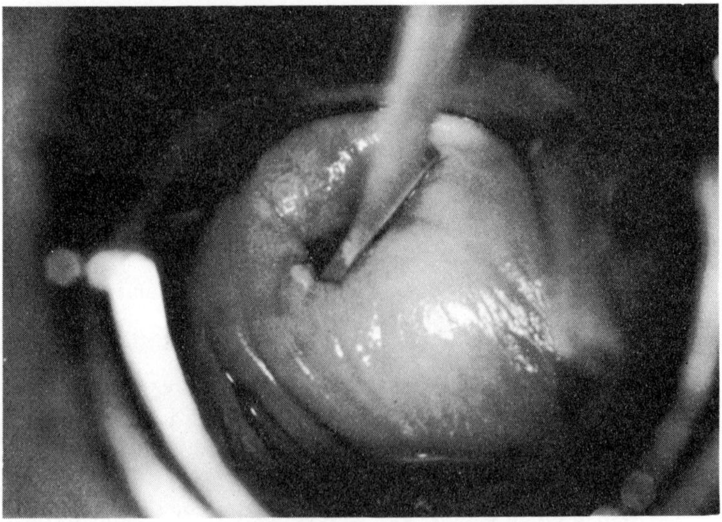

Fig. 3.1 Visualization of the entire cervix

Table 3.1 Causes of false positive cervical smears

Genital atrophy
Trichomonas vaginalis infection
Previous radiotherapy
Folic acid deficiency
Defective fixation
Defective smear identification
Laboratory errors

Table 3.2 Causes of false negative cervical smears

Smear not taken from the TZ
Too few cells on the slide
Smear covered with blood or pus cells
Excessive keratinization on the cervix
Defective fixation
Defective smear identification
Laboratory errors

cervix is slightly patulous but can be taken at any time provided no heavy bleeding is present.

Where an obvious macroscopic lesion is present a biopsy is preferable to a cytological smear.

Causes of false positive and false negative smears are listed in Tables 3.1 and 3.2.

COST OF SCREENING

The cost of mass screening is difficult to calculate; however, much attention has been drawn recently to the so called 'false negative' and inadequate smears which cause disillusionment among both healthcare workers and patients alike. Suggested causes are:

1. Inadequate training of cytotechnologists, cyto-pathologists and the sample taker.
2. Inadequacy of cytologic sampling due to poor sampling devices.
3. Inadequate time for examination of smears.

Inadequate sampling has led to the development of a plethora of new sampling devices. Until recently a cervical smear was pronounced 'unrepresentative' if it did not contain columnar endocervical cells, as the best results in detection of precancerous changes in the cervix depend on adequate sampling of the transformation zone. However, metaplasia of columnar cells to squamous epithelium occurs in this zone, often extending into the endocervical canal. The presence of endocervical columnar cells, metaplastic squamous cells, immature metaplastic and cervical mucous may reflect a well taken smear – provided the cellular material is plentiful and well preserved.

New sampling devices are too expensive for mass screening project in a Third World setting. Trials of these devices are costly and time consuming. A study of figures from this laboratory during the years 1987–1990 inclusive showed that a total of 299 287 smears were processed. The vast majority of smears were taken with the inexpensive Ayre spatula. Overall the detection of cervical dysplasia was not influenced by the presence or absence of endocervical cells as most dysplastic cells exfoliate readily. Also a high percentage of smears with no endocervical cells are taken from (1) pregnant patients, (2) post-menopausal patients, and (3) nulliparous women. This is due to the inaccessibility of the squamocolumnar junction. Tables 3.3 and 3.4 show the pick-up rate of CIN 2 and 3 in women in the above mentioned groups without endocervical cells on their smears during

Table 3.3 Lack of endocervical cells in patients with CIN

Specific Groups	*Total*	*Endocervical cells*		
		With	*Without*	*(%)*
Pregnant with CIN 2 or CIN 3	459	134	275	(60)
Over 50 years of age with CIN 2 or CIN 3	281	152	129	(45)
Nulliparous with CIN 2 or CIN 3	362	205	157	(43)

Table 3.4 Unrepresentative smears in specific groups of patients with suspicious or malignant lesions

		Endocervical cells	
	Total	*With*	*Without (%)*
Pregnant with suspicious or malignant	26	15	11 (42)
Over 50 years of age with suspicious or malignant	464	223	241 (52)
Nulliparous with suspicious or malignant	745	375	370 (49)

the years 1987–1990 inclusive. Approximately half of these patients had a significant abnormality detected on what would formerly have been considered 'unrepresentative smears'. The Ayre spatula yields representative smears, is inexpensive and easily available.

At Groote Schuur Hospital a total of 949 981 smears from women of all ages were examined during 1979–1992. There has been little change in the number of invasive cancers detected on smears because cervical smears are not usually taken in cases of clinically obvious neoplasms. The object of cervical smears is to detect occult, symptomless, preinvasive and microinvasive lesions. Comment can only be made on the increase in lesions per 1000 smears examined, as the exact population figures are unknown. Over the period 1988–1992 (5 years) 381 768 smears were screened in this laboratory. Of these, 75.9% were received from women between the ages of 20 and 40 years. During the 14 year period 1979–1992, the increase in CIN and HPV is graphically depicted in Fig. 3.2.

Follow-up varied from 63% in 1982 to 70% in 1992. Factors affecting follow-up are civil unrest, hospital strikes and closures associated with disruption of social, municipal and postal services.

Until recently it was taught that cervical neoplasia was a disease of middle aged women (more than 50 years of age). However, analysis of statistics during the years 1987–1992 inclusive, showed a peak incidence of CIN 2 and 3 in the 30–39 year age group.

TEENAGERS

In developing countries sexual activity appears to begin at an early age, thus leading to an increased incidence of abnormal cervical smears in teenagers. Worldwide there has been an increased focus on the problem of abnormal smears in young women (i.e. 19 years and younger). A rate of 15.2% abnormal smears in teenagers was reported

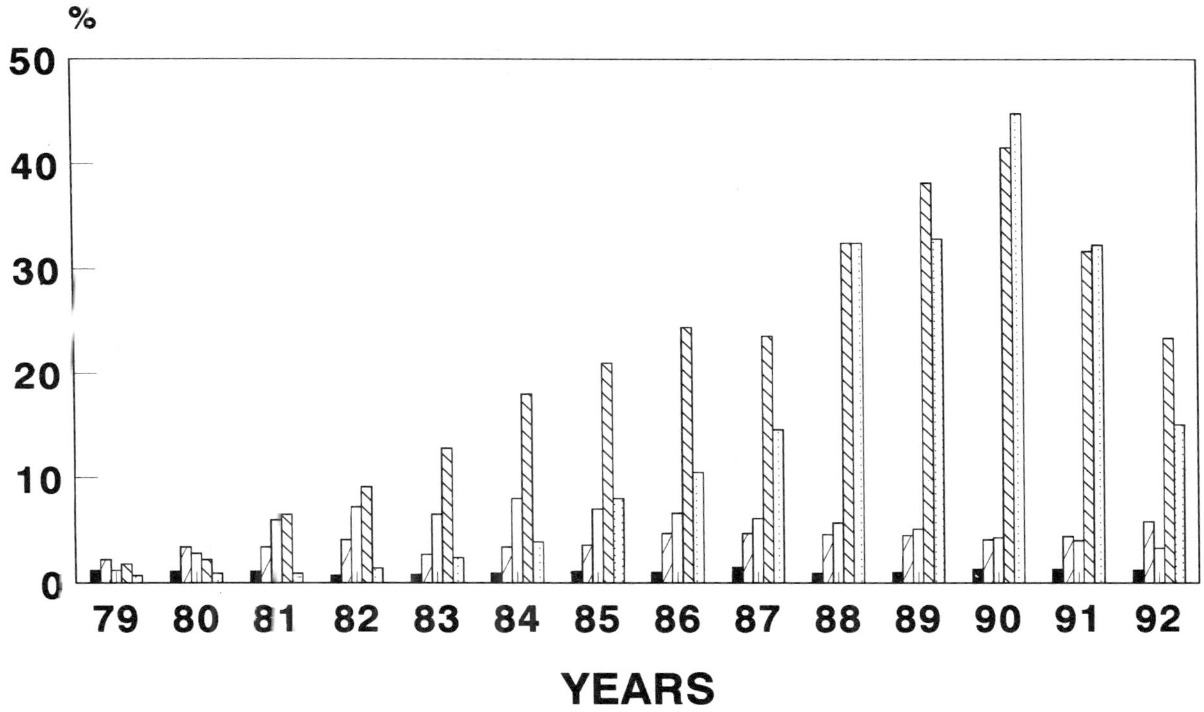

Fig. 3.2 Incidence of invasive squamous carcinoma (■) CIN 1 (▨), CIN 2 (□), CIN 3 (▧) and HPV (▒) over the 14-year period 1979–1992.

from this unit in 1990. A very high percentage of these teenagers were pregnant (84%). The figures are, however, biased as a Papanicolaou smear is routinely taken at their antenatal booking visit, while non-pregnant, sexually active teenagers do not usually have smears.

OLDER WOMEN

There seems to be a universal feeling that older women do not need cervical smears. However, the dysplastic process if it is already in progress does not suddenly stop in the 60th year. Figures from this unit show that there is a dire need to provide easy access to cervical screening for older women. During the period 1982–1992 inclusive, 11% of all patients with CIN 3 were from women over 50 years of age.

All of the above findings indicate that there is a great need for national cervical screening in a developing country.

In a developing country with rapid urbanization follow-up of patients with abnormal smears is difficult; however, with well-motivated staff, good record keeping and close liaison with community-based staff, good follow-up is possible.

Local cultural beliefs and traditions may prevent women from availing themselves of a screening service. However, if a service is free and readily available the local population is usually more inclined to use it. Mobile clinics would be an excellent way to reach these women and the possibility of treating patients at the time of diagnosis is being explored. An intensive educational drive is needed, through the medium of radio and national television if all population groups are to be reached.

ALTERNATIVE METHODS OF EARLY DETECTION OR SCREENING FOR CERVICAL CANCER

The establishment of a screening program in a country with a high incidence of preinvasive and invasive cervical cancer is unquestionably cost-effective but nevertheless enormously expensive. For this reason alternative options have emerged in the past decade.

1. Downstaging by visual inspection of the cervix. A cost-effective method with the major disadvantage that only invasive lesions are detected. Preinvasive lesions are very infrequently diagnosed. Little training and instrumentation are required, a biopsy is taken from the abnormal area, but preinvasive and HPV infections will be missed. The possibility of combining this method with acetic acid

staining holds promise of greater sensitivity and specificity and would in theory allow the early detection of preinvasive CIN.

2. Routine ablation of the transformation zone in the postpartum period has been investigated and an impressive study has demonstrated remarkable results with only 2 of 108 000 patients developing invasive cancer subsequently. This is basically a form of prophylaxis and has the obvious major disadvantage that large numbers of women are subjected to a painful unnecessary procedure.
3. Colposcopic screening is an option but has the obvious disadvantage of expensive equipment and training requirements. Biopsies are required in up to 15% of patients examined.
4. HPV:DNA screening, automated screening and the development of a vaccine against HPV are all being investigated at present and hold promise for the future.

4

Cytology of gynecological neoplasms

J. Whittaker

INTRODUCTION

The aim of this chapter is to briefly discuss and illustrate those tumors of the female genital tract and their precursor lesions which may be successfully diagnosed cytologically.

With the introduction of the cytological (Papanicolaou) smear as a meaningful diagnostic test in the 1950s, the reduction in incidence of squamous carcinoma of the uterine cervix has been repeatedly demonstrated and firm criteria have been established for the cytological diagnosis of squamous precursor lesions. The emphasis of this chapter will therefore be on these criteria, but as the scope of diagnostic cytology now extends beyond the confines of cervical squamous cell lesions a limited discussion will be given of other tumors of both the lower and upper genital tract.

VULVA

Vulval exfoliative cytology unfortunately cannot be used as a substitute for biopsy in the interpretation of vulval neoplasms as very vigorous scraping may be required to dislodge thick superficial layers of keratin and even then due to the frequent well-differentiated nature of vulval squamous carcinomas, the differentiation from *in situ* and precursor lesions may not be possible.

Similar problems may be encountered in the separation of pure vulval dystrophy from vulval intraepithelial neoplasia. Hyperkeratosis with parakeratosis may be the only abnormal cytological feature encountered in these vulval scrapes. However, the more severe the degree of dysplasia the more likely there are to be cells showing significant variation in nuclear size and shape, with hyperchromasia, on the smear.

Paget's disease of the vulva, melanoma and basal cell carcinoma have been diagnosed cytologically but again diagnosis of underlying invasive lesions and depth of invasion necessitate biopsy.

VAGINA

Primary malignant neoplasms of the vagina are extremely uncommon. Intraepithelial neoplastic lesions are also less common than their counterparts in the cervix but because the majority of preinvasive vaginal neoplasms are clinically silent cytology remains the most effective method of detecting these changes, particularly postradiation for cervical or intrauterine neoplasms. This raises the issue of differentiation of postradiation dysplasia from radiation-induced atypia which is a not infrequent problem encountered by the cytologist. Anisonucleosis and nuclear enlargement alone do not warrant the diagnosis of dysplasia as hyperchromasia, in particular, is required before this diagnosis can be made.

Clear cell carcinomas in young women and vaginal adenosis following DES exposure *in utero* are now rarely encountered but cytological follow-up of patients with vaginal adenosis has been suggested in the past as a screening method. Sarcomas, in particular botryoid rhabdomyosarcoma in children, may be diagnosed cytologically, particularly with the introduction of immunocytochemistry and electron microscopy into the realm of cytology. These methods, however, require sophisticated laboratory facilities.

UTERINE CERVIX

Squamous carcinoma and its precursor lesions

Precursor lesions of squamous carcinoma have been variously called dyskariosis, dysplasia, carcinoma *in situ*, cervical intraepithelial neoplasia and most recently in the Bethesda System squamous intraepithelial lesions of low and high grade. It is not the purpose of this chapter to discuss the various terminologic options but only to stress that failure to understand the clinical meaning of the cytopathologic evaluation may lead to inappropriate management. Perhaps the most widely used terminology remains cervical intraepithelial neoplasia (CIN) which is graded from 1 to 3. It has always been recognized that a proportion of these lesions may progress in severity and eventually may become invasive. The implication of the CIN concept is that all patients with these abnormalities require close cytological follow-up and if necessary colposcopic evaluation.

Cytological grading

Cytological smears are evaluated using a number of criteria but the most important in the assessment of grade of CIN relate to nuclear morphology and relative nuclear area. The morphology of cell nuclei in cases of squamous intraepithelial neoplasia comprize a combination of:

- Hyperchromasia
- Irregular chromatin configuration
- Disproportionate enlargement
- Anisonucleosis
- Abnormalities of nucleoli.

Relative nuclear area assesses nuclear cytoplasmic ratio and the greater size of nuclei reflects reduced maturation of the cell. Thus relative nuclear area increases with the severity of the lesion (Fig. 4.1).

It is important to stress that the cytological diagnosis of CIN relies on adequacy of sampling. These lesions generally arise in the metaplastic epithelium of the transformation zone and so the smear without endocervical columnar cells or an adequate number of

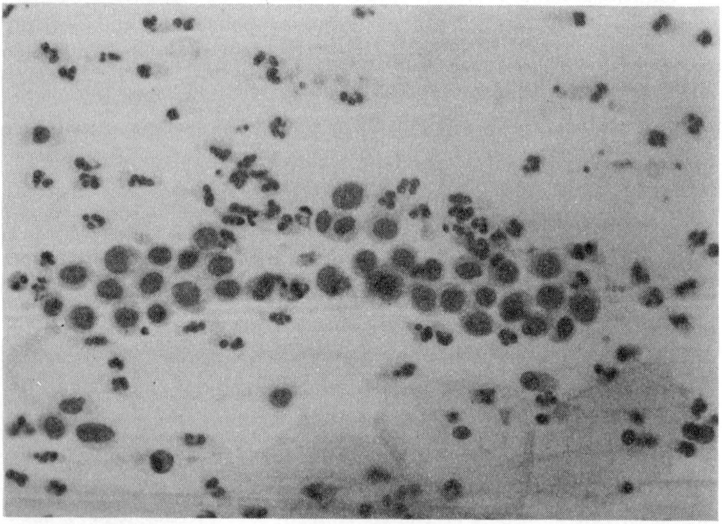

Fig. 4.1 Clusters of dysplastic cells showing nuclear irregularity, anisonucleosis, hyperchromasia and an increase in the nuclear/cytoplasmic ratio typical of CIN 2. Papanicolaou ×200.

metaplastic cells is less than optimal for cytological evaluation and false negative diagnoses may occur. Evaluation of heavily blood-stained smears and inflammatory smears may also be difficult as degeneration, in particular, distorts the morphology of cells.

Human papilloma virus

Certain subtypes of HPV have been implicated as etiologic agents of cervical carcinoma. Without specific immunohistochemical stains or *in situ* hybridization, specific subtypes cannot be recognized by cellular morphology alone. There are, however, certain features specific to all subtypes: these include koilocytosis, perinuclear haloing and dyskeratosis (abnormal cytoplasmic keratinization). These changes are often associated with CIN of all grades and the cytological diagnosis of HPV requires follow-up of the patient.

Squamous carcinoma

Cytologically, as well as histologically, three cell types are described; these include large cell keratinizing, large cell non-keratinizing and small cell squamous carcinoma. The cytological evaluation of these smears again includes nuclear morphology and relative nuclear area and these characteristics may resemble CIN 3. In addition, however, the smear background is 'dirty' as a result of tumor necrosis and hemolysis. The presence of a tumor diathesis in addition to clearly malignant cells with coarsely granular chromatin and nucleoli, is confirmatory cytological evidence of tumor invasion.

Keratinizing squamous carcinomas frequently contain elongated, cordate and bizarre cell forms with an orangeophilic keratinizing cytoplasm, as well as keratin pearls.

Small cell carcinoma is diagnosed when small cells with very hyperchromatic nuclei and little cytoplasm are seen on cytological smears.

Microinvasive carcinoma

Assessment of microinvasion by cytology alone may be difficult but features to note are the presence of prominent nucleoli in a smear which otherwise resembles CIN 3 and, in certain instances, highly atypical keratinization in a CIN 3 smear.

VERRUCOUS CARCINOMA

Verrucous carcinoma cannot be successfully diagnosed cytologically because of its bland cytological appearance and clinicopathological correlation is necessary.

ADENOCARCINOMA OF THE CERVIX AND ITS PRECURSOR LESIONS

Precursor lesions of adenocarcinoma

Adenocarcinoma *in situ* (AIS) and endocervical glandular dysplasia are the terms used for these lesions. The three main subtypes of AIS may on occasion also be recognized cytologically but the main criteria used for the cytological diagnosis of AIS pertain to the architectural features of endocervical glandular cells. These cells are seen as tightly crowded sheets in which there are gland openings and rosettes. Loss of polarity at the periphery of these sheets with 'feathering' is a particularly important cytological feature.

Endocervical glandular dysplasia is not easily recognized cytologically but essentially shows some but not all of the features of AIS. Its significance, in terms of progression, has not been adequately documented.

Adenocarcinoma of the cervix

The cytological classification of cervical adenocarcinoma is essentially the same as the histological classification but in the majority of instances the simple division of well differentiated from poorly differentiated forms is all that is possible. Degree of differentiation is graded on the basis of nuclear appearance. Smear background is not as useful a feature as with squamous carcinomas as a tumor diathesis is only infrequently found with invasive adenocarcinoma. The arrangement of the malignant cells is of paramount importance in the cytological diagnosis of adenocarcinoma. In addition to those features seen in AIS, supercrowding of nuclei is seen and singly lying malignant cells with nucleoli are often present (Fig. 4.2).

Adenosquamous carcinoma

These tumors would need to contain both squamous and glandular elements cytologically to be recognized as mixed tumors. Not in-

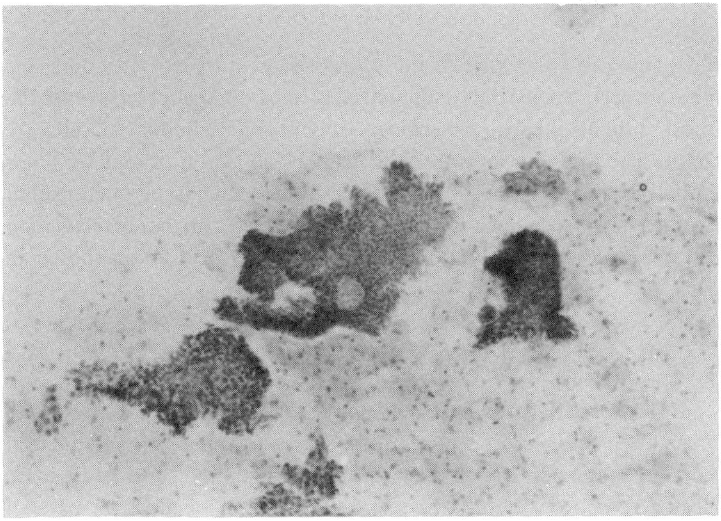

Fig. 4.2 Numerous crowded hypercellular groups of endocervical cells with peripheral feathering are cytologically typical of endocervical adenocarcinoma. Papanicolaou ×150.

frequently they are diagnosed as poorly differentiated carcinomas of either type.

PITFALLS IN THE DIAGNOSIS OF CERVICAL CANCER, PARTICULARLY IN DEVELOPING COUNTRIES

1. Atypical repair. Sheets of cells with prominent nucleoli are frequently seen associated with inflammatory conditions of the cervix. These changes may at times be difficult to differentiate from cervical neoplasms when there is in addition significant nuclear atypia.
2. Tuberculosis. Tuberculosis can occasionally involve the female genital tract and because of the associated necrosis of tissue with chronic inflammation may mimic carcinoma both clinically and cytologically. Recognition of granuloma formation is necessary for diagnosis and may not always be obvious on cytology.
3. Amoebiasis. Similar features to the above may be noted in cervical amoebomas; classical amoebae within the necrotic tissue may be difficult to identify.
4. Schistosomiasis. Extensive fibrosis and chronic inflammatory changes are the changes associated with schistosomiasis and again may mimic carcinoma cytologically and clinically. The ova occasionally may be found on cytology smears.

ENDOMETRIUM

Cytology can contribute to the diagnosis of endometrial tumors, including early lesions, but endometrial cytology probably represents the most difficult area in gynecological cytology. Endometrial cells are frequently present in routine Papanicolaou smear samples. Their appearance in smears from postmenopausal women or perimenopausal women in the second half of the cycle necessitates further investigation as a small number of endometrial carcinomas may be diagnosed in this way.

Direct sampling of the endometrium

A variety of different sampling devices have been used over the years in an attempt to provide an adequate screening device for endometrial carcinoma. Factors which may need to be taken into consideration are cost, acceptability to the patient and the provision of adequate material for evaluation. In addition to this, considerable experience is required for adequate cytologic interpretation.

ENDOMETRIAL CARCINOMA AND ITS PRECURSORS

Hyperplasia and atypical hyperplasia

The sampled fragments appear on the smears as sheets of surface endometrium, glandular structures and loose stromal cells. Interpretation of hyperplasia on an endometrial sample may be difficult but nuclear enlargement, crowding and prominence of nucleoli in glands are the features which are notable. If in addition there were anisonucleosis, atypical hyperplasia may be suspected.

Endometrial carcinoma

The amount of material obtained is variable but usually depends on the experience of the sampler as well as the intrinsic nature of the tumor. Recognition of loss of polarity as well as anisonucleosis in gland fragments is required for a cytological diagnosis of endometrial carcinoma. The cytological features, particularly of well-differentiated adenocarcinoma, are subtle but the more poorly differentiated the tumor the more pleomorphic it is and the more easily it is diagnosed cytologically (Fig. 4.3). A watery, granular tumor diathesis background is also frequently encountered with large, vacuolated histiocytes. Occasional psammoma bodies are identified which may be indicative of a papillary serous endometrial carcinoma.

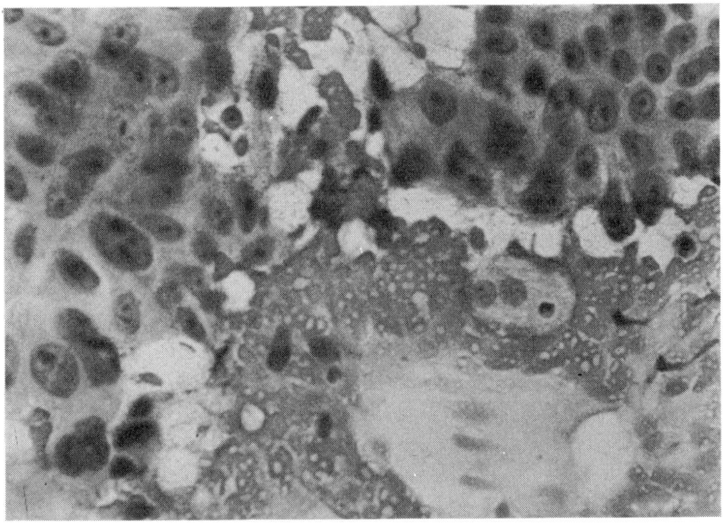

Fig. 4.3 Malignant cells directly sampled from the endometrium, using an endopap sampler, show prominent nucleoli as well as marked variation in nuclear size and shape. Note the background of hemolysed blood. Papanicolaou ×500.

With few exceptions it is difficult to diagnose cytologically specific cell types of adenocarcinoma of the endometrium. Usually the cellular features reflect the endometrial origin of the tumor and the changes of differentiation but not the specific histologic subtypes.

Endometrial stromal neoplasms are rare and the cytologic features are not well documented.

CARCINO SARCOMA (MALIGNANT MIXED MÜLLERIAN TUMOR)

Carcino sarcoma is usually diagnosed as being an adenocarcinoma cytologically as the superficial layers which are exfoliated are generally epithelial in type. Occasional spindle or strap-shaped cells may be present on the smear and if these are recognized the diagnosis of carcino sarcoma may be suggested.

MYOMETRIUM

Sampling devices are designed to sample superficial layers of the uterine cavity and for that reason uterine leiomyosarcomas are rarely diagnosed cytologically. Occasionally a submucosal leiomyoma, which is superficially ulcerated, may yield spindle-shaped cells containing cigar-shaped nuclei but this is an infrequent event.

DIAGNOSIS OF EXTRAUTERINE MALIGNANCY ON CERVICAL AND UTERINE SAMPLES

The ability to differentiate malignant cells of extrauterine origin from those of primary cervical or intrauterine origin is of importance as it may help to determine the nature of the investigation. Factors which may be important in influencing the shedding of malignant cells of extrauterine origin into the uterus, cervical canal or vagina include site of primary tumor, extent and location of neoplastic spread, ascites and fallopian tube involvement. Those cells exfoliated are usually poorly differentiated and degenerate but typically 'balled up' and are seen as three-dimensional clusters with a clearing effect around the cluster. Tumor diathesis is generally lacking and these two typical features help to differentiate primary from metastatic adenocarcinoma (Fig. 4.4).

Adenocarcinoma of the fallopian tube may have an associated watery diathesis.

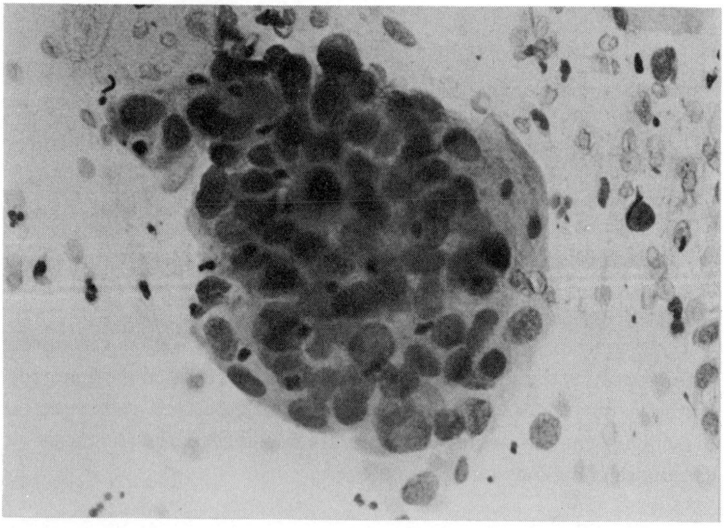

Fig. 4.4 Three-dimensional cluster of air dried glandular cells in a clean background as is seen with exfoliated malignant cells from the upper genital tract. Papanicolaou ×500.

Serous carcinoma of the ovary may exfoliate with psammoma bodies, which would suggest ovarian origin.

Of course tumors from the gastrointestinal tract or metastatic tumors from other sites, in particular the breast, may shed cells in a similar fashion and may be diagnosed in this way.

OVARIAN TUMORS

Although benign ovarian cysts may be successfully aspirated and diagnosed cytologically, the place of cytology in the diagnosis of ovarian tumors is limited and generally this diagnosis is not made by direct sampling. It is not recommended that fine needles be inserted into suspected ovarian neoplasms either transabdominally or by colpo puncture as the seeding of malignant cells into the peritoneal cavity is to be avoided.

Malignant cells may however exfoliate down into the lower genital tract, as discussed, or in the presence of associated ascites malignant cells may be recognized in the serous fluid.

CYTOLOGY OF ASCITIC FLUID

The number of neoplastic cells is usually high with the cells presenting as large acinar or papillary clusters mixed with singly lying cells. The papillary clusters may contain psammoma bodies. These features strongly suggest ovarian origin but other metastatic adenocarcinomas may show similar features. Pseudomyxoma peritonei may also be diagnosed cytologically, classically with sparse well-differentiated mucin-producing cells in a myxoid background.

5

Stoma care in gynecological cancer

P. Stevens

INTRODUCTION

The prospect of undergoing formation of an intestinal stoma is still a daunting one, even in the face of skilled and supportive stomal nursing care, empathic surgeons and advanced technology. This is especially so for patients from a poor socioeconomic and educational background. Culturally, acceptance of a stoma is still a problem area. Time, simplistic explanation and rationalization need expert explanation. Further to this, many patients cannot make a decision of such magnitude without consulting with other family members. This is a problem when such a family is not in close proximity to the hospital. To embark on stomal surgery without them being involved in the preparatory stage may make life for the patient subsequently untenable.

In gynecological cancer there are four groups of patients that may require intestinal diversion.

1. Those with advanced disease requiring palliative diversion.
2. Those with invasion of the bowel or urinary tract by tumor requiring temporary or permanent diversion as part of the tumor removal procedure.
3. Those with postradiation injury to bowel or urinary tract who may require single or double diversion.
4. Stomatherapy techniques may also be required in the management of draining wounds and fistulae.

The key to successful stoma surgery and rehabilitation lies both in impeccable surgical technique and in the provision of adequate emotional and practical support for patient and family. All patients undergoing stoma construction, either as an elective or emergency procedure, require the service of an informed stomatherapy nurse as part of the multidisciplinary team. The role of the nurse includes the provision of preoperative counseling and orientation, stomal siting, postoperative practical management and education, discharge planning and ongoing community and outpatient clinic care.

PREOPERATIVE COUNSELING AND ORIENTATION

Patients come from a wide range of social, cultural and religious backgrounds and each requires an individualized approach, also involving a close family member or friend. Orientation methods include education on the normal anatomy and physiology of the gastrointestinal or genitourinary tract, with a simplistic description of the passage of food and liquid between mouth and anus or kidney and urethra. By utilizing models and diagrams it is possible to delineate the part of the anatomy compromized by disease or injury and demonstrate the surgical plan and the site of the fecal or urinary diversion. When indicated, the prospective stoma patient may benefit from meeting a well-matched rehabilitated ostomate with a similar stoma, condition and social background. Questions and concerns regarding sexuality, diet, prognosis and lifestyle should be openly discussed. An introduction to simplistic pouching and skin care and the knowledge that ongoing practical care and support will be available following discharge from hospital go far in helping a patient to accept the prospect of an intestinal diversion.

STOMA SITING

This aspect of preoperative preparation is vital to the success of the procedure! A poorly placed stoma can lead to leakage, odor, skin breakdown and a host of emotive and psychosocial problems. To achieve the ideal site acceptable to both patient and surgeon, the patient must be examined in the lying, sitting and standing position in order to note the changing body contours.

Criteria for siting intestinal stomas

The chosen site should avoid:

- Costal margins
- Waistline
- Umbilicus
- Surgical incision
- Obvious abdominal folds and creases

- Scars
- Anterior iliac crests.

Utilize a skin protective wafer with a central hole and place on the proposed site to ensure the skin surface covered does not encroach on the wound or umbilicus. Once satisfied, mark the site with a skin pen.

SPECIAL CONSIDERATIONS

1. Obese patients. Note the pendulous abdomen in the standing position; place a site where the patient can see the stoma and ensure it is marked on the summit of any fat folds.
2. Patients for radiotherapy. When radiotherapy is planned in pelvic or intra-abdominal malignancy, place the stoma in a lateral site and higher on the anterior abdominal wall to avoid as much of the radiation field as possible. **Adhere to the criteria for all stoma siting** – keep the stoma within the rectus abdominis muscle.
3. Wheelchair-bound patients and orthopedic/neurologic pathology. Site the patient in the wheelchair or wearing any braces or external appliance to ensure the site does not encroach or compromise. Note any scoliosis or kyphosis and place the stoma in the most convenient site for patient self-management. This may mean siting on the opposite side to the conventional.

PRACTICAL MANAGEMENT OF FECAL STOMAS

A wide range of products exist for the practical management of intestinal stomas.

1. Pouches. Ostomy pouches are plastic, odor-proof and disposable. They can be opaque or non-opaque, closed or drainable, one or two piece. The adhesive materials are variable with the majority being hypo-allergenic. Closed pouches are ideal for ostomates with a well-formed stool and are removed once or twice daily. Drainable pouches are left in place for as long as they are leak-proof and comfortable, usually 3–5 days, and the stool is drained from the pouch using a releasing clip. Two-piece equipment enables the adhesive base to be left in place and either a closed or drainable pouch affixed as required. This system is ideal in patients with very sensitive skin or in those receiving radiotherapy, as the base can be cut back and the pouch angled away from the treatment area. With postoperative pouching it is advisable to utilize a drainable system with peristomal skin protection until the stool pattern is firmly established.

2. Flatus patches. Many of the closed-type colostomy pouches have a built-in charcoal flatus patch allowing flatus to be spontaneously filtered and deodorized. Patches can also be affixed to pouches but should not be placed on drainable pouches as they only remain odor-proof for approximately 24 hours.
3. Skin protective wafers. Skin protective wafers are made from pectin and carboxymethyl cellulose. Their function is to protect skin from the adhesive of pouches and to provide a firm base as additional security.
4. Stoma pastes. Pastes are utilized as fillers when irregular skin surfaces compromise continence. Spirit within the paste compounds may cause a temporary stinging sensation when applied to raw skin.
5. Stoma powders. Stoma powders are ideal for insufflating onto traumatized or bleeding stomal mucosa. The powder forms a protective gel until healing takes place. It may also be lightly dusted onto broken skin.
6. Convex inserts and convex faceplates/one piece convexity pouches. These are utilized to promote a 'pouting' of flush stomas, especially when ileal diversions or ileostomies have not been adequately fashioned as a spout.
7. Belts. The majority of drainable and urinary pouches provide an integral belting system for use in extreme activity or to provide added security, especially in difficult or high output ostomates.

STOMAL COMPLICATIONS

Dermatologic

The most common causes of sore skin are:

1. Fecal contamination. Especially effluent from the ileum and right-sided colostomies. The usual reason for this occurring is application of the wrong diameter pouch, allowing feces in contact with peristomal skin for a prolonged period of time or leaking equipment due either to poor application, poor siting or surgical construction. Retracted stomas with resulting skin creases require intensive stoma care or, on occasions, reconstruction or re-siting.
2. Allergy to the adhesive of the pouch or adhesive tape. An obvious distribution of the erythematous or excoriated skin will give the clue to this distressing condition. Immediate removal of the offending adhesive and application of a protective skin wafer with a one or two-piece pouching system usually rapidly clears the problem. The offending adhesive may be found in several of the available

pouches; in highly sensitive cases, two-piece equipment with no other adhesive than that of a methyl cellulose wafer will solve the problem.

3. Fungal and/or bacterial infections. High out-put stomas with leakage onto the skin can present a major management problem. Should fungal overgrowth occur, dermatologic opinion should be sought and the use of topical anti-fungal and anti-inflammatory agents are sometimes prescribed. The problems of adherence of equipment is maximal when any topical ointment is required. The use of a belt will give added security.
4. Mechanical trauma. Patients who usually have formed stools and wear closed pouches remove their pouch once or twice daily. More frequent removal of any type of pouch will result in a damaged epidermis. Drainable pouches either of a one or two-piece variety should be recommended to all patients with frequent stooling habits.

Surgical complications

- Paracolostomy hernia
- Prolapse
- Retraction
- Peristomal granulation – stomal granulations
- Stenosis
- Bolus obstruction
- Stomal separation – peristomal sepsis
- Ischemia.

STOMAL FUNCTION

This is governed by the following factors:

- Physical status
- Dietary habits
- Level of the stoma within the gastrointestinal tract
- Surgery performed (short circuit of gut or resection)
- Medications (analgesics, antibiotics, chemotherapy)
- Radiation sequelae.

DIARRHEA

First principles include the provision of drainable pouches with adequate skin protection. Adequate hydration with oral or intravenous replacement. 'Blockers' such as Imodium (loperamide), codeine phosphate or Lomotil or the use of 'bulkers' such as bran, Metamucil, Normacol should only be used if the patient is known to have no narrowed segments of small or large bowel secondary to disease or radiation fibrosis. Bolus obstruction can occur in such cases.

CONSTIPATION

This problem is very prevalent in patients with poor appetite and regular analgesic ingestion. Such patients should be on a preventative regular aperient and stool softener. Should they become impacted or 'obstipated', a lactulose aperient such as Duphalac or sorbitol is recommended. To relieve a frankly 'obstipated' stoma, gentle instillation of warm olive oil via the stoma is recommended. This may be accomplished by inserting a catheter past the impacted fecal bolus and slowly instilling the oil over a 20 minute period. The patient should also be given a stat dose of oral castor oil (150 ml). If the stool does not move spontaneously over the following 12 hours, a gentle colostomy wash-out utilizing a colostomy wash-out set should be carried out.

Having cleared the bowel of feces, high fluid intake and adequate fiber coupled with a regular softener and propellant will prevent further problems.

PSYCHOLOGIC COMPLICATIONS

The very nature of the precipitating condition, unpleasant symptoms and complications leading to diversion all give ample reason for depression. The loss of sexuality, rejection and loss of support from loved ones are further compounded by an onslaught on their body image. Ongoing and regular support for patient and partner is required to gain acceptance. This reactive depression improves in the majority of cases without medication or psychiatric intervention.

FISTULAE

In approximately 48% of stage 4 cervical carcinoma patients, invasion of the urinary tract will result in fistulae or obstruction. The unpleasant symptoms are such that if a prognosis of several weeks is predicted, palliative diversion will assist the remaining quality of life. When a shorter prognosis is predicted, palliation by provision of suitably absorbent pads and panties with skin protection and hygiene by vulval swabbing at regular intervals are indicated. A further technique of containing the fistula efflux is to insert a vaginal catheter and collect the urine in either a bedside bag or, if the patient can be mobilized, leg bag.

Stoma care for fistulae

1. Clean and dry the skin around the stoma.
2. 'Pipe' stoma paste around the cutaneal opening as a washer.
3. Apply a pouch of a drainable or 'urostomy' type to the skin ensuring that the opening of the pouch is cut to leave no skin exposed to the effluent.

Simple method of managing vesico–vaginal fistulae by a vaginal plug and catheter

REQUIREMENTS

- A 20 ml syringe (with the top cut off)
- A condom or the finger of a surgical glove
- Silicone liquid and the activator
- Remicaine jelly
- Foley's catheter or argyle tubing
- Urinary leg bag or bedside urinary bag
- Sanitary towel.

METHOD

Add the activator to the silicone and stir until thick. Remove the plunger and insert the liquid silicone into the syringe and put the same into the glove or condom. Lubricate liberally and insert into the vagina. Depress the plunger and leave the silicone *in situ* for 5–10 minutes. Leave it to dry but do not allow to get totally so. Pull the foley or argyle tubing through the centre of the prosthesis with a pair of mosquito forceps. Once the prosthesis is completely dry – insert into the vagina, cut a small hole in a sanitary towel and pass the tubing through it. The foley can then be placed onto drainage via either leg or bedside urinary drainage bag.

This same method may be utilized to relieve enterovaginal fistulae. While not always entirely effective, it is a method that can alleviate unpleasant symptoms effectively either temporarily or even permanently.

INTESTINAL URINARY DIVERSIONS

Formal urinary diversion utilizing either ileum or colon are called urostomies. The resultant urinary stoma is made as a spout everted stoma rather than a flush intestinal stoma to ensure easy collection of urine into a urostomy pouch. Flush stomas lead to problems with pooling of urine, phosphate burns to the stomal mucosa and eventually to stenosis of the stoma.

POUCHING

Urinary pouches may be one or two-piece systems. They all have a tap mechanism to facilitate drainage of the urine without pouch removal. This in turn can be connected to a bedside urine bag to enable daily monitoring of the inpatient output and to enable the home urostomate to get a good night's rest.

LONG-TERM MANAGEMENT

Regular assessment of urinary stomas is vital if complications are to be avoided.

1. Simple digital examination of the stoma to assess any cutaneal or deep rectul stenosis. Urine pooling in the stoma will lead to urinary tract infection.
2. Bacteriologic examination of urine sampled directly from the conduit via a sterile catheter should be performed if the patient is symptomatic.
3. Ultrasound of the kidneys annually after diversion. Should hydronephrosis be detected, a conduitogram will assess the ureteroileal anastomosis for possible stenosis.

MANAGEMENT OF MALIGNANT ASCITES UTILIZING THE BELFORT DRAINAGE METHOD

Ascites is a common complication in patients with advanced malignant disease. It is usually very disabling and this justifies active intervention.

THE BELFORT UCT DRAIN

A new approach to the problem of managing intractable malignant pre-terminal ascites has been made by a team from Groote Schuur

Hospital, Cape Town. They have devised an intra-abdominal silastic drain with an external tube with a self-operated clamp. This enables the patient to drain ascites as often as required on a daily or twice daily basis. It is specifically designed to drain thick proteinaceous fluid and can be flushed if patency is compromized.

1. Orientation of patient and family. This is an important aspect and should be performed prior to using the drain.
2. Siting the drain. In advanced malignancy, an ultrasound is performed to elicit the best spot for drain insertion to achieve maximum benefit. Many cases have marked loculations of fluid; thus unplanned placement may result in poor drainage.
3. Drain insertion. Following local anesthetic infiltration, a small transverse incision is made through the left or right rectus muscle into the peritoneal cavity. The drain is inserted and a purse-string suture placed around the Dacron cuff of the tube within the rectus muscle. The smaller bore to be exteriorized is tunneled via the abdominal wall to a convenient site approximately 5 cm from the incision. The tube is clamped by the closure mechanism. Once the skin incision has been closed, a two-piece urostomy system (e.g. 45 mm Squibb Convatec System two or four) is applied over the external drain. The sutured wound will be under the base of the system, covered with a light non-adherent dressing.
4. Two-piece urostomy drainage system. The rationale for using this type of system is to promote a 'closed system' that allows drainage without frequent handling in a controlled fashion. The operator is able to release the clamp of the external tube by depressing the clamp through the bag.

REALISTIC DILEMMAS

Each potential ostomy patient requires a careful holistic approach and it is in the light of both a full medical and social assessment that the ultimate decision will be made. The difficulties in decision making are usually those surrounding lack of family support, practical available assistance and the possible lack of adequate ostomy supplies.

Family support

This is especially necessary in patients with advanced disease who may continue to manifest lower abdominal and vaginal symptoms, such as pain and discharge, and may require assistance in the correct application of pouches. The fear of having a member of the family with bowel exteriorized upon the skin and emitting feces, often results in eviction from the dwelling unless adequate counseling and support can be given by professionals.

To go without a pouch is out of the question, as skin problems and odor only compound the situation and will have done little to give any quality of life.

Centers providing stoma advice and equipment

Sadly, the costs of both stomatherapy-trained personnel and equipment involve large sums of money. Thus, many patients in Third World scenarios undergoing stomal surgery experience severe hardship from lack of appropriate equipment and informed personnel to help them if complications of a dermatologic or functional nature occur. It has been the objective of our service to provide such personnel and equipment at suitably-based key hospitals throughout the country, each in turn linking with small centers, and providing the equipment required for the individual patients having their surgery at major centers and then returning home. This is a major financial undertaking and a problem that faces even the most established first world centers worldwide. In our hands, it requires a dedicated team at the base hospital to ensure that the equipment is provided and reaches the correct patient 'up country'. Ambulance services, farm lorries and willing volunteers traveling to distant areas provide the means of transport. It is 'sub optimal' in as much as little individualized ongoing support is given but at least the efflux is contained.

The question is, should one embark on stomal surgery without the appropriate equipment to provide an odor-proof, trouble-free life for the patient? There is no comprehensive answer. If at the very least equipment can be provided and the patients taught how to care for themselves adequately prior to discharge, then an ongoing hospital supply is a viable option. If this cannot be guaranteed, stomal construction should be avoided. Individual circumstances will ultimately dictate the appropriate measures.

6

Premalignant lesions of the vulva, vagina and cervix

B. Lindeque

PREMALIGNANT LESIONS OF THE VULVA

Premalignant squamous cell lesions

The histopathologic descriptive terminology of intraepithelial lesions of the vulva has been the subject of numerous revisions and classifications and it is likely that more will follow. Furthermore, differing terminologies are used in various parts of the world. In this chapter **vulvar intraepithelial neoplasia (VIN)** grade 3 will be used to indicate carcinoma *in situ* and its histopathological equivalents. Using this classification, VIN 1 will indicate squamous dystrophic vulvar lesions with mild atypia and VIN 2 lesions moderate atypia.

ETIOLOGY

The etiology of VIN 3 is not known. Neither the herpes simplex virus type 2 (HSV-2) nor the human papilloma virus (HPV) have been convincingly implicated as the cause of VIN 3. The presence in VIN 3 lesions of HPV particles has, however, been demonstrated by immunoperoxidase staining and *in situ* hybridization.

The most important associations of VIN 3 are with cervical intraepithelial neoplasia (35%) vaginal intraepithelial neoplasia (12%), condylomata acuminata (>50%), invasive carcinomas of the cervix (2%) and vulva (up to 18%). Infrequently, a patient may present with VIN 3, vaginal intraepithelial neoplasia and cervical intraepithelial neoplasia. This has become known as the 'lower genital tract neoplasia syndrome'. Associated HPV infection is frequently present and this disorder is indicative of the 'field' effect of genital carcinogenesis.

CLINICAL PROFILE

VIN 3 has in the past been regarded as an uncommon disease occurring in postmenopausal women. In recent years the incidence has increased significantly (Fig. 6.1) and younger women are affected. The mean age currently is 35–40 years.

At least 50% of patients are asymptomatic. If symptoms do occur, pruritus, burning or the presence of nodules on the vulvar skin are the most common manifestations. The classical VIN 3 lesion is a raised hyperpigmented lesion, often with central red and white (depigmented) areas. Lesions are multicentric in two-thirds of cases and may be discrete or coalescent. The distribution of lesions and frequency of site involvement is shown in Fig. 6.2.

DIAGNOSIS

Careful inspection of the vulva remains the most important diagnostic technique followed by colposcopy with a 3% acetic acid solution.

The diagnosis must be confirmed by biopsy. In the case of small or localized lesions, this is an easy office procedure under local anesthesia. Most patients have multicentric lesions requiring multiple biopsies of all affected areas which are best taken under general anesthesia. Vulvar biopsies should be deep enough to include all skin layers.

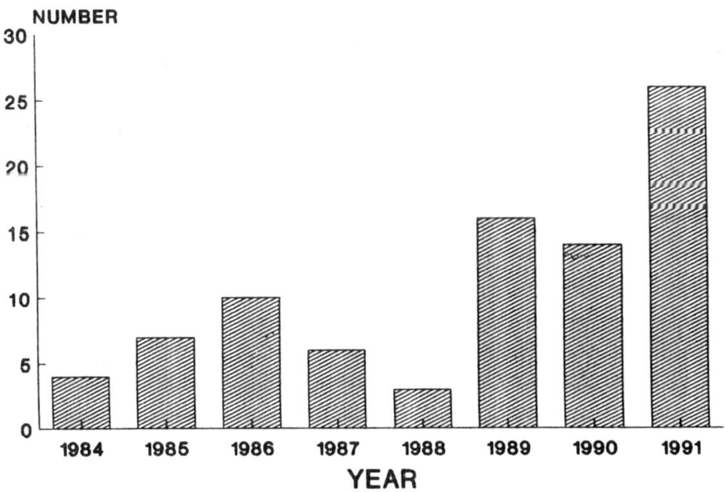

Fig. 6.1 New cases of VIN 3 seen at the University of Pretoria Academic Hospitals.

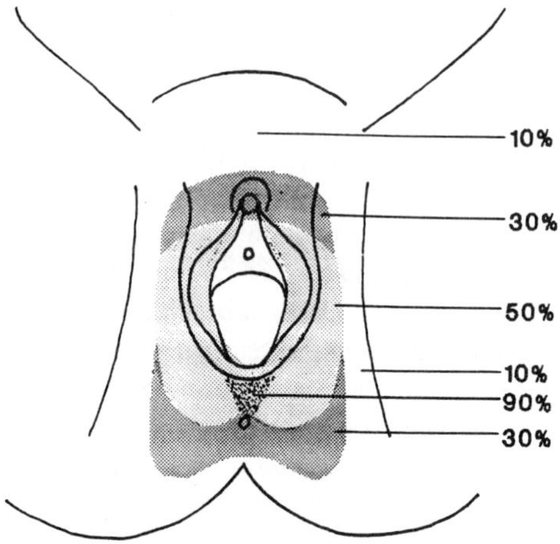

Fig. 6.2 Distribution of VIN lesions.

TREATMENT

Treatment of VIN 3 is influenced by the extent of the lesion. Small unifocal lesions can be removed by excisional biopsy. Multifocal lesions can be treated with CO_2 laser. This procedure will require general anesthesia. The surgeon must be experienced in laser surgery and must possess knowledge of the technique. A recurrence rate of up to 20% emphasizes the importance of regular follow-up.

Partial skinning vulvectomy is an excellent alternative method of managing multifocal VIN 3. The clitoris can almost always be preserved and, even if involved, the epithelium can be scraped from the glans and a further advantage is that VIN 3 is occult in about 19% of cases. The recurrence rate is also around 20%.

Topical 5-fluorouracil has been used to treat VIN 3 with some success but should only be used where other more effective treatment modalities are contraindicated.

PROGNOSIS

VIN 3 is regarded as a disease with a low malignant potential and an excellent prognosis. This is not uniformly true and progression to invasion occurs in 1–4% of cases.

Paget's disease of the vulva

Extramammary Paget's disease has recently been classified as non-squamous VIN and is a rare disease. The lesion is red with white scales and is frequently well demarcated. Extreme pruritus is a common symptom. The disease may be multicentric and can extend beyond the visible borders of the lesion.

Treatment is by excisional biopsy or partial vulvectomy.

Up to 26% of patients may have another non-contiguous malignant lesion. The most common sites are the cervix, breast, rectum and bladder.

PREMALIGNANT LESIONS OF THE VAGINA

Areas of vaginal intraepithelial neoplasia (VaIN) in association with cervical intraepithelial neoplasia occur in 4–6% of cases. The occurrence of VaIN in the vaginal vault following hysterectomy is also a problematic condition.

Most, but not all, patients with VaIN of the vaginal vault have previously had CIN which suggests a shared etiology. It is usually asymptomatic and the presence of VaIN is detected on vaginal vault cytology. Colposcopy should be performed and acetowhite patches identified. The entire vagina must be examined, especially the vaginal vault angles.

Occult invasive carcinoma has been reported in 28% of patients with VaIN-positive cytology. The treatment of choice for the post-hysterectomy patient is excision or laser ablation if proven non-invasive on histology.

Annual cytologic vault smears for follow-up and early detection of VaIN are essential where the indication for a prior hysterectomy was CIN.

PREMALIGNANT LESIONS OF THE CERVIX

Cervical cancer is the most common malignancy in South African women accounting for 32.7% of all cancers. A well-planned cytologic population screening program is essential to reduce the incidence of this preventable disease.

Premalignant squamous lesions: cervical intraepithelial neoplasia (CIN)

EPIDEMIOLOGY OF CERVICAL SQUAMOUS CELL NEOPLASIA (CHAPTER 1)

TRANSFORMATION ZONE

After puberty, the original squamocolumnar junction migrates outwards on the ectocervix forming a physiologic ectopy. Concurrently, mainly due to a decrease in the vaginal pH, the exposed endocervical cells undergo squamous metaplasia, thus forming the transformation zone (TZ). The metaplastic squamous epithelium joins the endocervical columnar epithelium at a new squamocolumnar junction (SCJ). If, at the time of metaplastic transformation, the patient is exposed to one or more carcinogens, an abnormal dysplastic TZ is formed. Such a dysplastic TZ forms a 'carcinogenic field' containing one or more foci of atypical cells. These foci eventually overcome local host defence mechanisms, increase in number and replace normal cells. This results in the formation of CIN lesions which may have malignant potential. The position of the SCJ is not static and relocates with changes in estrogen levels. During pregnancy, the SCJ migrates widely out on the ectocervix. Small positional changes may take place during the normal menstrual cycle and with the use of hormonal contraceptives. In the perimenopause and climacteric, the SCJ migrates upward into the endocervical canal.

CLASSIFICATION AND NATURAL HISTORY OF CIN

Currently the following histopathologic classification of cervical intraepithelial neoplasia is in general use with subdivision into the three grades of CIN 1, CIN 2 and CIN 3. It is thought that most lesions start as CIN 1 and either persist, regress or progress to CIN 2 and then CIN 3.

It is unlikely that CIN 2 and CIN 3 lesions will regress. The annual incidence of cervical carcinoma in patients with CIN 3 is approximately 1650 per 100000 and in untreated CIN 3, more than 20% of patients will develop invasive carcinoma within 20 years.

Persistent squamous cell atypia has a progression risk to CIN 2–3 of 16–37%. Cervical HPV lesions may regress spontaneously, persist for long periods but about 30% of such lesions will progress to CIN within 6–18 months.

Recently, a new classification system for cervical premalignant lesions was proposed (the Bethesda System) using the term squamous intraepithelial lesion (SIL). This is subdivided into SIL, low grade (equivalent to atypia, CIN 1 and HPV) and SIL, high grade (equivalent to CIN 2 and 3 and HPV with CIN). It was proposed that the Bethesda classification replaces the Papanicolaou grading system and it has gained acceptance in many cytology and histopathology laboratories with debatable pros and cons. For clarity the Papanicolaou system will be used in this text.

DETECTION OF CIN: CYTOLOGY

The typical patient with CIN is asymptomatic and between 20 and 30 years of age. Rarely postcoital bleeding is noted. Cervical cytology fulfills all the requirements of an ideal screening test (see Fig. 6.3).

Smears indicating squamous atypia, HPV infection or CIN 1 should be repeated after 6 months. If the same grade of abnormality persists for two or three smears, referral for colposcopy is indicated. The risk for occult CIN 3 in such patients may be as high as 60%.

Smears indicative of CIN 2, CIN 3, CIN with HPV and of possible invasive carcinoma are indications for immediate action.

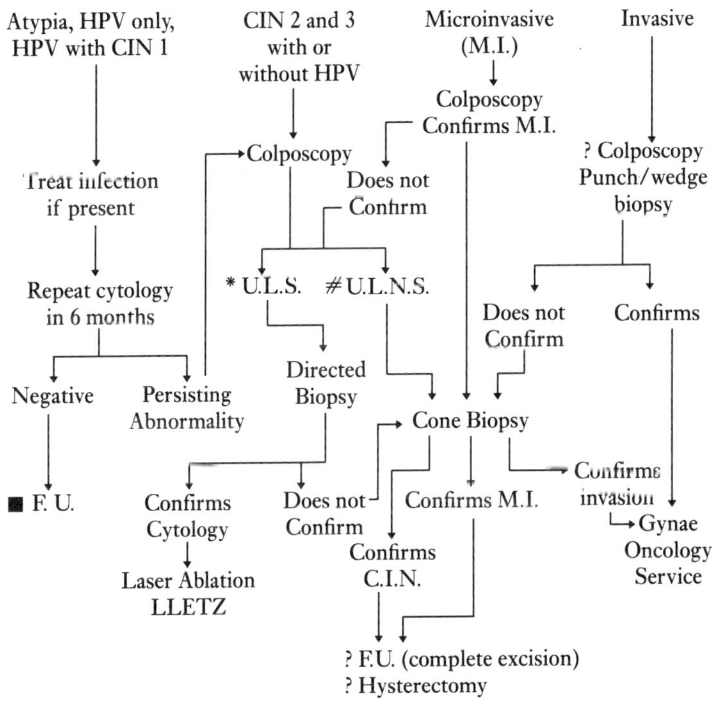

* Upper Limit of abnormal area seen
# Upper Limit of abnormal area not seen
■ F.U. = Follow up: suggested 6 monthly cytology for 3 years then annually

Fig. 6.3 Management of the patient with an abnormal smear.

COLPOSCOPY

As cytology is a screening test, the final diagnosis is made histologically on a cervical biopsy. The use of the colposcope allows the clinician to examine the cervix under magnification and with the use of 3% acetic acid and iodine as staining agents to take a directed biopsy. The colposcopist must ensure that the entire TZ is visualized (satisfactory colposcopy). The colposcopic parameters indicative of CIN are acetowhite epithelium, mosaic or punctation patterns and abnormal blood vessels (Figs 6.4–6.6).

Biopsies are to be taken from the most abnormal areas. With satisfactory colposcopy, the predictive value of the directed biopsies is excellent. If colposcopy is unsatisfactory, biopsies are not reliable and a diagnostic cone biopsy is indicated.

CONE BIOPSY

The current indications for cone biopsy include:

1. Cytology showing CIN 2, CIN 3 or HPV with CIN, where colposcopy is not available.
2. Unsatisfactory colposcopy: where the entire TZ is not visible.
3. Where colposcopically-directed biopsies show a lower grade of abnormality than the cytology and colposcopy.

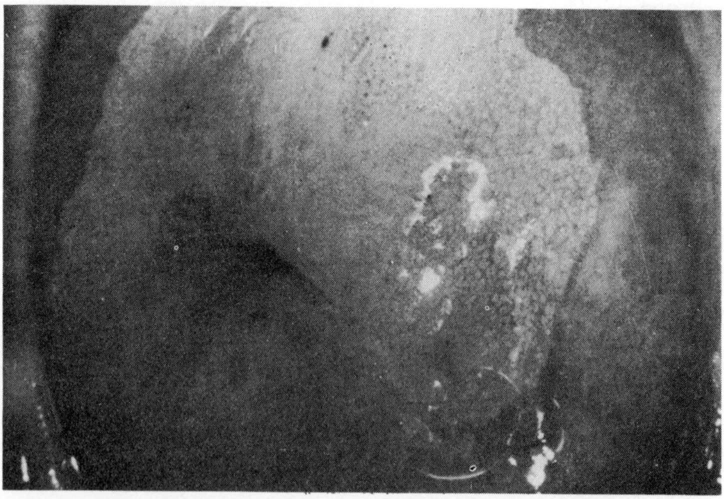

Fig. 6.4 Colposcopical photograph of the cervix showing acetowhite epithelium and mosaic pattern.

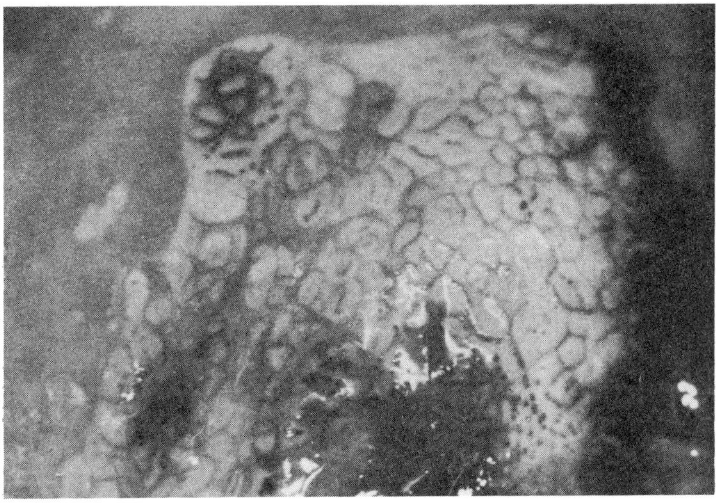

Fig. 6.5 Close-up colposcopical photograph of the cervix showing punctation and mosaic pattern.

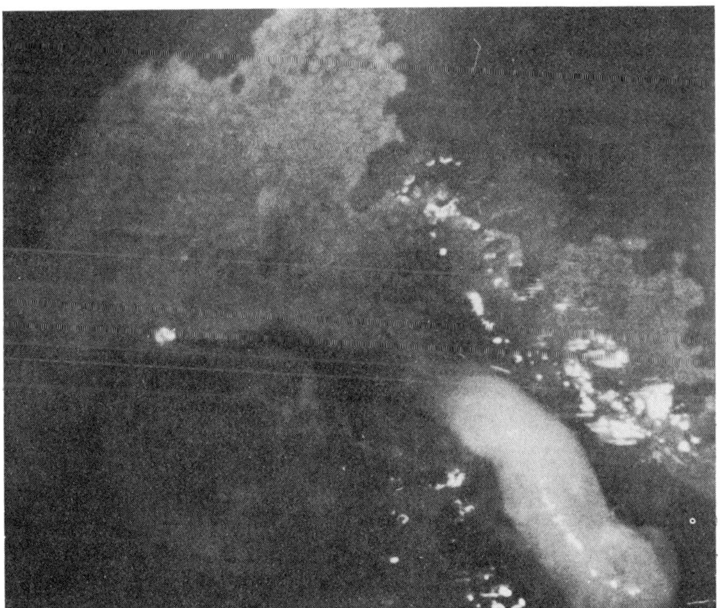

Fig. 6.6 Colposcopical photograph of the cervix showing acetowhite epithelium and mosaic pattern. Note the irregular outline suggestive of HPV infection.

4. Where the directed biopsy indicates microinvasive carcinoma, this is necessary to exclude invasive cancer.
5. Where endocervical adenocarcinoma is suspected.
6. Rarely, where cone biopsy is used as a primary therapeutic procedure.

Cone biopsy carries a major risk of morbidity and many complications, including infertility due to excision of gland-bearing portions of the cervix, cervical stenosis or incompetence. It should not be used, therefore, in young patients as a primary procedure. Cone biopsy will, however, be necessary in many patients over 35–40 years of age with CIN 2 or CIN 3 because of the endocervical position of the SCJ.

Laser conization offers an attractive alternative to cold knife cone biopsy, especially in young women.

Recently the use of cone biopsy for unsatisfactory colposcopy in the atypia/CIN 1 cytology groups has been questioned as the incidence of negative cone biopsies was found to be 64%. It is recommended that patients with the above be biopsied if colposcopically-visible lesions are present, despite the colposcopy being unsatisfactory, and that an endocervical brushing or curettage should be performed.

MANAGEMENT OF CIN

The options are:

1. Local destructive therapy.
   (a) CO_2 laser: success rate 95%.
   (b) Cryotherapy: success rate 80%.
   (c) Radical deep cautery: success rate 90%.
   (d) LLETZ: success rate 95%.
2. Hysterectomy: abdominal or vaginal.

Follow-up 6 monthly for 3 years, then annually.

LLETZ (large loop excision of the transformation zone) was introduced as a therapeutic option in 1989. A thin wire loop is used to excize the transformation zone using electrodiathermy, and the bed is cauterized. Several studies have now confirmed that this method allows for excellent histopathology and rapid, single-visit office therapy with a recurrence rate of CIN of 2–5% after 6–12 months. Long-term results are still awaited. LLETZ has been used since February 1991 at Kalafong Hospital, University of Pretoria. Due to the relatively low cost of the diathermy equipment required and the advantages of single-visit therapy, this method may be ideally suited for use in developing countries. A major problem in such countries when dealing with CIN is the lack of successful recall. Despite all efforts to trace and recall patients, only 80% of patients with abnormal smears at Kalafong Hospital, University of Pretoria, were successfully traced in 1991. In many hospitals this figure is lower.

CIN IN PREGNANCY

These patients are usually young and treatment should be as shown in Fig. 6.7.

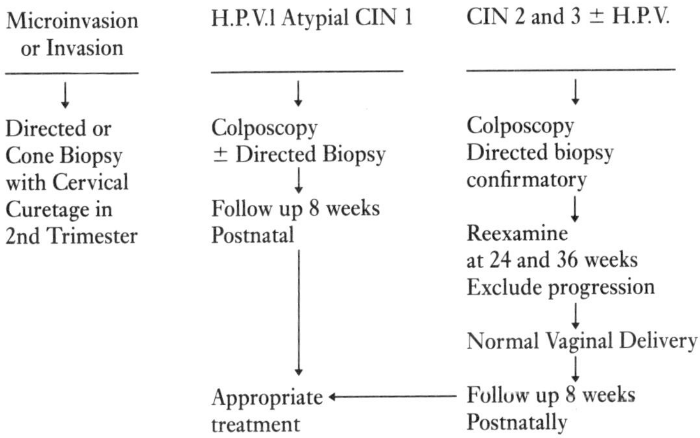

Fig. 6.7 Treatment of patients with CIN in pregnancy.

Cervical adenocarcinoma *in situ*

Adenocarcinoma *in situ* (AIS) of the cervix is uncommon. It may be the only abnormality but in two-thirds of cases there is associated CIN. It is usually asymptomatic but may present with abnormal vaginal bleeding or a blood-stained vaginal discharge. The typical patient is in her fifth decade, parous and although the epidemiologic features associated with CIN are usually absent, an association between AIS and HPV type 18 has been suggested.

Due to its endocervical location, colposcopy is of limited value in further evaluation but endocervical brushing may alert the clinician.

The treatment modalities most commonly used are hysterectomy or cone biopsy. A recurrence rate of 5–7% has been reported.

7

Staging procedures for gynecological cancers

J. Knobel

The staging procedures recommended by the International Federation of Gynecology and Obstetrics (FIGO) should be adhered to. Since 1966 the TNM Committee of the International Union Against Cancer (UICC) has made recommendations regarding staging and classification of gynecological tumors. At present the FIGO and TNM classifications are in full conformity with each other.

CANCER OF THE CERVIX

Rules of staging

1. Clinical staging. The primary staging procedure is clinical. Clinical examination should be performed by an experienced examiner. Although anesthesia is recommended for this examination, it is not practical where large numbers of new cases are seen and staged.

   The following examinations are permitted: inspection, palpation, colposcopy, endocervical curettage, hysteroscopy, cystoscopy, proctoscopy, intravenous urography, barium enema and X-ray examination of the lungs and skeleton. Other examinations like computerized tomography are optional but the findings should not be the basis for changing the clinical staging.

   (a) The initial clinical staging should not be changed because of subsequent findings.

   (b) When there is doubt about the stage, the earlier stage should be reported.

   (c) Institutions in developing countries manage many patients with cervical cancer. Under these circumstances it is time and cost-effective to dispense with intravenous pyelography and to diagnose hydronephrosis and hydroureter sonographically. Similarly, skeletal metastases are diagnosed better by radioactive whole body scan than by radiological skeletal survey.

However, in the developing world cost-effective investigating is required and for practical purposes the latter investigation can be dispensed with because of low yield. At present these modifications are not accepted by FIGO if statistics are to be reported for inclusion in the 'Annual Report on the Results of Treatment in Carcinoma of the Uterus, Vagina and Ovary', which is a voluntary collection and collaboration of data.

2. Surgical evaluative staging. Conization or amputation of the cervix is regarded as a clinical examination. Invasive cancers diagnosed in this way are included in the statistics.
3. Pathologic staging. Pathologic examination of surgically removed tissue can accurately assess the extent of disease. These findings cannot change the clinical staging but should be reported separately.

Staging classification (FIGO nomenclature)

Stage 0	Carcinoma *in situ*, intraepithelial carcinoma (not included in the therapeutic statistics.
Stage I	The carcinoma is strictly confined to the cervix (extension to the corpus should be disregarded).
Stage Ia	Preclinical carcinoma of the cervix: i.e. those diagnosed only by microscopy.
Stage Ia(i)	Minimal microscopically evident stromal invasion.
Stage Ia(ii)	Lesions detected microscopically that can be measured; the upper limit of the measurement should not show a depth of invasion of more than 5 mm taken from the base of the epithelium, either surface or glandular, from which it originates and a second dimension (the horizontal spread) must not exceed 7 mm; larger lesions should be staged as Ib.
Stage Ib	Lesions of greater dimension than stage Ia(ii) whether seen clinically or not; preformed space involvement should be specifically recorded so as to determine whether it should affect treatment decisions in the future.
Stage II	The carcinoma extends beyond the cervix but has not extended to the pelvic wall. The carcinoma involves the vagina but not as far as the lower third.
Stage IIa	No obvious parametrial involvement.
Stage IIb	Obvious parametrial involvement.
Stage III	The carcinoma has extended to the pelvic wall. On rectal examination there is no cancer-free space between the

	tumor and the pelvic wall. The tumor involves the lower third of the vagina. All cases with hydronephrosis or non-functioning kidney are included unless they are known to be due to another cause.
Stage IIIa	No extension to the pelvic wall.
Stage IIIb	Extension to the pelvic wall and/or hydronephrosis or non-functioning kidney.
Stage IV	The carcinoma has extended beyond the true pelvis or has clinically involved the mucosa of the bladder or rectum. A bullous edema as such does not permit a case to be allotted to stage IV.
Stage IVa	Spread of the growth to adjacent organs.
Stage IVb	Spread to distant organs.

Notes about staging

1. Stage 0 comprises those cases with full thickness involvement of the epithelium with atypical cells but with no signs of invasion into the stroma.
2. Stage Ia should include minimal microscopically-evident stromal invasion as well as small tumors of measurable size; therefore lesions with minute foci of invasion visible only microscopically as Ia(i) and the macroscopically measurable microcarcinoma as stage Ia(ii). The term Ib occult should be omitted.
3. The diagnosis of both stage Ia(i) and Ia(ii) should be based on microscopic examination of removed tissue, preferably a cone, which must include the entire lesion. The lower limit of stage Ia2 should be that which can be measured macroscopically (even if dots need to be placed on the slide before measurement) and the upper limit of Ia2 is given by measurement of the two largest dimensions in any given section. The depth of invasion should not be more than 5 mm taken from the base of the epithelium, either surface or glandular, from which it originates. The second dimension, the horizontal spread, must not exceed 7 mm. Vascular space involvement, either venous or lymphatic, should not alter the staging but should be specifically recorded.
4. It is impossible to estimate clinically if cervical cancer has extended to the corpus uteri. Extension to the corpus should therefore be disregarded.
5. The presence of bullous edema as such does not permit a case to be allotted to stage IV. Malignant cells on cytology from the bladder require a biospy from the bladder wall.

CANCER OF THE ENDOMETRIUM

It has been recognized for some time that certain factors are prognostically significant in endometrial carcinoma. Those factors are:

- Stage of the disease
- Histologic type
  - endometroid adenocarcinoma
  - adenosquamous carcinoma
  - clear cell carcinoma
  - serous papillary carcinoma
  - undifferentiated carcinoma
- Histologic grading
  - 1: well differentiated
  - 2: moderately differentiated
  - 3: poorly differentiated
- Depth of myometrial invasion
- Lymph–vascular space invasion
- Peritoneal cytology
- Pelvic and/or para-aortic lymph node metastases.

The recognition of the significance of these factors led FIGO to change the staging of endometrial carcinoma from clinical to surgical. The initial examination is clinical, aimed at recording an initial staging to facilitate planning of the subsequent surgical procedure. The staging is only finalized after histopathologic examination of surgically removed tissue. The current FIGO staging for endometrial carcinoma is as follows:

FIGO (1988) staging of endometrial carcinoma

Stage Ia G1, 2 or 3	Tumor limited to the endometrium
Stage Ib G1, 2 or 3	Invasion to inner half of the myometrium.
Stage Ic G1, 2 or 3	Invasion to outer half of the myometrium.
Stage IIa G1, 2 or 3	Endocervical glandular involvement only.
Stage IIb G1, 2 or 3	Cervical stromal involvement.
Stage IIIa G1, 2 or 3	Tumor invades the uterine serosa and/or the adnexa and/or positive peritoneal cytology.
Stage IIIb G1, 2 or 3	Vaginal metastases.
Stage IIIc G1, 2 or 3	Metastases to pelvic and/or paraaortic lymph nodes.
Stage IVa G1, 2 or 3	Tumor invasion of bladder and/or bowel mucosa.

Stage IVb Distant metastases including intra abdominal and/or inguinal lymph nodes.

Histopathology: degree of differentiation

G1 5% or less of a non-squamous or non-morular solid growth pattern.
G2 6–50% of a non-squamous or non-morular solid growth pattern.
G3 More than 50% of a non-squamous or non-morular solid growth pattern.

Notes regarding staging

1. The inclusion of three important prognostic factors in the staging procedure is to be welcomed (histologic grading, depth of myometrial invasion and occult involvement of the cervix). Certain controversial aspects remain, e.g. the high staging value of positive peritoneal cytology (stage IIIa), the inclusion of retroperitoneal lymph node dissection (which is a formidable procedure if done fully in obese, often medically unfit, elderly patients) and the fact that lymph–vascular space invasion is disregarded in the staging.
2. Because endometrial carcinoma is now staged surgically some procedures previously used for determination of stages such as fractional dilatation and curettage are no longer applicable.
3. There may be a small number of patients treated primarily by radiation therapy. In such cases the clinical staging adopted by FIGO in 1971 would still apply but the use of that staging system should be noted.
4. Ideally, the width of the myometrium should be measured as well as the depth of the tumor invasion.
5. In subgrouping cases according to the degree of differentiation described on microscopic examination, the predominant lesion is adenocarcinoma but all histologic types should be recorded. However, choriocarcinomas, sarcomas, mixed mesodermal tumors and carcinosarcomas should be presented separately.

CANCER OF THE OVARY

Ovarian malignancies are staged according to the FIGO system described in 1987. This staging is based on the findings at surgical exploration. Preoperative assessment should exclude the presence of extraperitoneal metastases. The importance of thorough surgical staging cannot be overemphasized because subsequent treatment will be determined by the stage of disease.

This involves the following steps after the abdomen is opened by a midline or paramedian incision:

1. Any free fluid, especially in the pouch of Douglas, should be retrieved and submitted for cytologic assessment. Cytologic smears should also be made and fixed in theater.
2. Peritoneal lavage should be performed and specimens obtained from the pouch of Douglas, each paracolic gutter and gauze wipes from beneath each hemidiaphragm.
3. A systematic exploration of all the intra-abdominal surfaces and viscera is performed, proceeding clockwise from the cecum along the right paracolic gutter and ascending colon, right kidney, liver, gallbladder, right hemidiaphragm, entrance to the lesser sac, along the transverse colon to the left hemidiaphragm, left kidney and down the left paracolic gutter and descending colon to the sigmoid colon and rectum. The entire small bowel with its mesentery should be inspected carefully.
4. Any suspicious areas or adhesions should be biopsied. If no evidence of disease is found, biopsies of the peritoneum of the pouch of Douglas, both paracolic gutters and the uterovesical pouch should be taken.
5. An infracolic omentectomy is performed.
6. Any enlarged lymph nodes are resected and submitted separately for histopathologic assessment. Nodal tissue is sampled from the external and internal iliac vessels, the common iliac, the obturator fossa and the paraortic area.

Carcinoma of the ovary: staging using the FIGO nomenclature

Stage I	Growth limited to the ovaries.
Stage Ia	Growth limited to one ovary, no ascites; no tumor on the external surface; capsule intact.
Stage Ib	Growth limited to both ovaries; no ascites containing malignant cells; no tumor on the external surfaces; capsules intact.
Stage Ic	*Tumor either stage Ia or Ib but with tumor on the surface of one or both ovaries; or with capsule ruptured; or with ascites present containing malignant cells or with positive peritoneal washings.

Stage II	Growth involving one or both ovaries with pelvic extension.
Stage IIa	Extension and/or metastases to the uterus and/or tubes.
Stage IIb	Extension to other pelvic tissues.
Stage IIc	*Tumor either stage IIa or stage IIb but with tumor on the surface of one or both ovaries; or with capsule(s) ruptured; or with ascites present containing malignant cells or with positive peritoneal washings.
Stage III	Tumor involving one or both ovaries with peritoneal implants outside the pelvis and/or positive retroperitoneal or inguinal nodes; superficial liver metastases equals stage III; tumor is limited to the true pelvis but with histologically-verified malignant extension to small bowel or omentum.
Stage IIIa	Tumor grossly limited to the true pelvis with negative nodes but with histologically-confirmed microscopic seeding of abdominal peritoneal surfaces.
Stage IIIb	Tumor of one or both ovaries; histologically-confirmed implants of abdominal peritoneal surfaces, none exceeding 2 cm in diameter; nodes negative.
Stage IIIc	Abdominal implants greater than 2 cm in diameter and/or positive retroperitoneal or inguinal nodes.
Stage IV	Growth involving one or both ovaries with distant metastases; if pleural effusion is present, there must be positive cytology to allot a case to stage IV; parenchymal liver metastases equals stage IV.

* If possible, it should be recorded if rupture of the capsule was (1) spontaneous, or (2) caused by the surgeon and if the source of the malignant cells detected was peritoneal washings or ascites.

CANCER OF THE VULVA

A clinical staging system based on the TNM classification was adopted by FIGO in 1969. This staging is based on a clinical evaluation of the primary tumor and regional lymph nodes and a limited search for distant metastases.

Clinical staging of carcinoma of the vulva

T:	*Primary tumor*
T1	Tumor confined to the vulva, 2 cm in largest diameter
T2	Tumor confined to the vulva, >2 cm in diameter

T3 Tumor of any size with adjacent spread to the urethra and/or vagina and/or perineum and/or anus

T4 Tumor of any size infiltrating the bladder mucosa and/or the rectal mucosa or including the upper part of the urethral mucosa and/or fixed to the bone

N: *Regional lymph nodes*

N0 No nodes palpable

N1 Nodes palpable in either groin, mobile, not clinically suspicious for neoplasm

N2 Nodes palpable in either or both groins, enlarged, firm and mobile, clinically suspicious for neoplasm

N3 Fixed or ulcerated nodes

M: *Distant metastases*

M0 No clinical metastases

M1 Palpable deep pelvic lymph nodes

M1b Other distant metastases

FIGO stage: clinical findings

Stage 0 Carcinoma *in situ*, e.g. VIN 3

Stage I Tumor confined to the vulva, 2 cm or less in largest diameter and no suspicious groin nodes.

Stage II Tumor confined to the vulva, more than 2 cm in diameter and no suspicious groin nodes.

Stage III Tumor of any size with: adjacent spread to the urethra and/or the vagina, the perineum and the anus and/or clinically suspicious lymph nodes in either groin.

Stage IV Tumor of any size: infiltrating the bladder mucosa or the rectal mucosa or both, including the upper part of the urethral mucosa and/or fixed to the bone and/or other distant metastases.

Clinical evaluation of the groin lymph nodes is inaccurate in about 25% of cases. When compared with surgical staging the error in clinical staging is about 20% for stage I disease and about 40% for stage IV disease.

A new FIGO staging for vulval cancer, based on surgical findings, was adopted at the 1988 FIGO meeting in Rio de Janeiro, Brazil.

Stage I Tumor confined to vulva or perineum, 2 cm less in diameter.

Stage II Tumor confined to vulva or perineum, more than 2 cm in greatest dimension.

Stage III	Tumor of any size that invades any of the following: lower urethra, vagina, anus and/or unilateral lymph node metastases.
Stage IVa	Tumor invades any of the following: upper urethra, bladder or rectal mucosa, pelvic bone and/or bilateral regional lymph node metastases.
Stage IVb	Distant metastases.

CANCER OF THE VAGINA

The rules for staging carcinoma of the vagina are similar to those for the cervix.

Staging classification (FIGO nomenclature)

Stage 0	Carcinoma *in situ*; intraepithelial carcinoma.
Stage I	The carcinoma is limited to the vaginal wall.
Stage II	The carcinoma has involved the subvaginal tissue but has not extended to the pelvic wall.
Stage III	The carcinoma has extended to the pelvic wall.
Stage IV	The carcinoma has extended beyond the true pelvis or has involved the mucosa of the bladder or rectum; bullous edema as such does not permit a case to be allotted to stage IV.
Stage IVa	Spread of the growth to adjacent organs and/or direct extension beyond the true pelvis.
Stage IVb	Spread to distant organs.

CANCER OF THE FALLOPIAN TUBES

There is no official FIGO staging for tubal cancer but the ovarian staging system has been adapted to apply to fallopian tube disease. Staging should therefore be according to the surgical findings.

Surgical staging of carcinoma of the fallopian tubes

Stage I	Carcinoma confined to fallopian tube(s).
Stage Ia	Unilateral disease; no ascites.
Stage Ib	Bilateral disease; no ascites.
Stage Ic	Either Ia or Ib with ascites and/or malignant cells in peritoneal washings.

Stage II	Carcinoma extends beyond fallopian tube(s) but is confined to the pelvis.
Stage IIa	Extension to uterus and/or ovary.
Stage IIb	Extension to other pelvic organs.
Stage IIc	Either IIa or IIb with ascites and/or malignant cells in peritoneal washings.
Stage III	Carcinoma extends beyond the pelvis but is confined to the abdominal cavity.
Stage IIIa	Microscopic tumor only.
Stage IIIb	Tumor diameter 2 cm or less.
Stage IIIc	Tumor diameter more than 2 cm and/or positive retroperitoneal or inguinal lymph nodes.
Stage IV	Carcinoma extends beyond abdominal cavity; if pleural effusion is present, there must be positive cytologic findings to allot the case to stage IV; parenchymal liver metastases equals stage IV.

CONCLUSIONS

The philosophy behind staging of these tumors is the following:

1. It allows for the adoption of treatment protocols in individual institutions.
2. It instills a disciplined and systematic approach to patients with gynecological cancer.
3. It allows assessment of results in individual institutions and also the implementation of randomized clinical trials.
4. It allows for comparison of results between institutions where protocols differ for various standardized disease stages.

8

Perioperative and operative management of gynecological cancers

B. Bloch

INTRODUCTION

The perioperative management of gynecological cancers is central to the successful outcome of any operation. In developing countries there are a number of considerations which are paramount and which are not usually operative in developed countries. These include the non-availability of social services, poor living conditions, poverty, nutritional deprivation and the lack of back-up services for patients with ostomies. Differing cultural beliefs and language difficulties may also bedevil communication and compliance.

Most procedures for gynecological cancer are elective and allow properly planned pre-, intra- and postoperative care. This, together with good clinical judgement in the selection of patients for surgery, will contribute significantly to a successful outcome for the individual patient.

PREOPERATIVE MANAGEMENT

Initial consultation

It is important to establish a good rapport with the patient at the first visit. Very often an interpreter is required to explain the nature of the problem and the solution available. An empathic approach to a nervous and frightened patient will go a long way towards reassuring an often bewildered person.

A full history and a complete clinical physical examination are essential. These will be followed by the appropriate basic investigations to establish the suspected diagnosis. These investigations may include:

- Biopsy
- Fine needle aspiration biopsy
- Sampling of the endometrium.

Certain routine investigations may also be performed at this time such as:

- Full blood count
- X-rays of the chest or abdomen
- Ultrasound where indicated on clinical or staging grounds
- Quantitation of urea, creatinine and electrolytes.

After any additional explanation and reassurance the patient should be scheduled for a second consultation where the results of the above investigations are available and the diagnosis established. Where doubt exists additional investigations are arranged.

Second or follow-up consultation

1. This is when the diagnosis is established.
2. A full explanation of the implications is essential.
3. Treatment options are discussed with all the relevant facts highlighted.
4. Further investigations are arranged to accurately stage the particular tumor. These may include:
   (a) Intravenous pyelography.
   (b) Cystoscopy.
   (c) Where chemotherapy is likely, e.g. trophoblastic tumors.
   (d) Tumor markers where indicated.
5. Testing for HIV positivity is becoming increasingly relevant in developing countries and if not performed routinely should be included where any clinical suspicion exists.
6. Specialized visualization techniques, such as tomography, CT scans or MRI are very seldom available and even if available contribute very little to staging of gynecological tumors.
7. Concurrent medical complications and diseases are assessed. The following are particularly important:
   (a) Diabetes.
   (b) Hypertension.
   (c) Morbid obesity.
   (d) Pulmonary status.
8. Infections: particularly tuberculosis, syphilis, HIV status, bilharzia, schistosomiasis.

9. Nutritional status must be assessed and if not adequate steps must be taken to correct any deficiencies.
10. Concurrent medication. This must be assessed and any alterations necessary made.
11. Consent for operation must be signed and the full extent of the envisaged procedure and the postoperative expectations must be explained in detail. This discussion should include answering any questions the patient may want to ask and questions should be encouraged in an attempt to allay the patient's real fears. Due to poor educational standards and language difficulties the validity of informed consent is sometimes questioned in developing countries. This fear can be allayed if a full explanation is given through an interpreter.

Immediate preoperative management

The following should be considered and instituted in the 24 hours immediately prior to surgery.

1. Bowel preparation. The simplest effective method should be used. Magnesium citrate in liquid form (200 ml) is given by mouth 18–24 hours prior to surgery. A low residue diet is commenced 1 day prior to this followed by a liquid diet until the nil per mouth period immediately preceding surgery. Older patients are particularly prone to develop oliguria postoperatively and adequate hydration should be ensured during the 24 hours preoperatively especially if the magnesium citrate causes diarrhea. Alternative more expensive preparations such as Golightly are available but have no advantages over magnesium citrate.
2. Vaginal preparation. Betadine douches are recommended and are given 24 and 12 hours preoperatively. No additional preparation is required.
3. Physiotherapy. All patients undergoing major gynecological cancer therapy have one or more risk factors for major complications. Physiotherapy including early mobilization to prevent the most feared of these complications (atelectasis, chest infections and deep venous thrombosis) is of prime importance. If a qualified physiotherapist is not available this can be effectively done by the medical and nursing staff using simple techniques.
4. Prophylactic antibiotics. Postoperative infection is a frequent complication of cancer surgery and antibiotics should be used judiciously. The best combinations will cover a broad spectrum and

in particular Gram-negative organisms and anaerobes. It is common practice to prescribe this type of prophylaxis for three doses given intravenously at 8 hourly intervals the first being administered 1 hour before surgery. Drugs commonly used in various combinations are high dose penicillin, metronidazole, gentamycin and the second or third generation cephalosporins. It should, however, be remembered that meticulous hemostasis and judicious drainage of wound sites will contribute more than antibiotics to the prevention of postoperative sepsis.

Pathogenic organisms vary from institution to institution and thus appropriate antibiotic regimens will also vary.

5. Prophylactic anticoagulation. This is recommended in association with physiotherapy and elastic stockings, if possible of the graduated pressure type, to prevent thromboembolic complications. Until recently, calcium heparin (5000–10 000 units) was given subcutaneously twice daily for 5–7 days postoperatively but this regimen has been replaced by enoxaparin at the dose of 40 mg daily given subcutaneously for the same period of time. The starting dose is given 12 hours preoperatively.
6. Frozen section histology. This may be important in deciding on the type and extent of the operative procedure and should be arranged if available and appropriate.

CARE IN THE OPERATING THEATER

Prior to anesthesia

The following important aspects must be attended to:

1. Positioning of the patient. The surgeon must ensure that this is optimal and in particular that there is no undue pressure on the lower legs. Simultaneously the position of the cautery electrodes must be checked.
2. Catheterization. Asepsis and antisepsis as well as meticulous technique are important and many surgeons prefer to do this personally. After completion, position of the catheter should be checked and in particular undue tension on the urethra should be avoided.
3. Vaginal preparation. This again should be meticulously performed using an antiseptic solution such as povidone-iodine or Hibitane. When vaginal plugging is required, such as prior to a radical hysterectomy, good technique is essential to ensure that the operator gains maximal advantage from the maneuver. The vagina should be tightly plugged from the cervix to the introitus.

4. Abdominal preparation. This is often taken for granted and not carried out properly. The umbilicus must be cleaned and an antiseptic solution applied from 'nipples to knees' to ensure good asepsis and antisepsis. Similarly, the draping of sterile towels must not be haphazard. A sterile technique is important for the prevention of infection.
5. Communication with colleagues. It is essential that the anesthetist is informed of the scope of the envisaged procedure not only preoperatively but kept informed during the procedure. Any concerns and in particular blood loss must be communicated. Before the blood pressure falls significantly, 25% of the blood volume must be lost. Blood volume is about 70 ml/kg and in a 65 kg female this loss will be 1140 ml. It is far better to have this fluid loss replaced immediately than to face the consequences postoperatively. Similarly, the scrub sister and other involved nursing staff must be kept involved and interested.

Intraoperative care

While it is not possible to describe in detail the important points relating to each procedure the following are important.

1. The incision. This should be adequate for the procedure. Individual surgeons will have their own preferences but it should be kept in mind that a basic principle of cancer surgery is adequate exposure. In the abdomen a full laparotomy for staging purposes is mandatory. This can most often only be achieved by a vertical incision which can if necessary be extended both up and downwards. Particularly in the management of ovarian cancer, the above is of paramount importance for the treatment depends on accurate staging and if carried out at the first operation will avoid repeat, often complex and dangerous surgery.
2. Tissue handling. Gentleness in handling tissues is paramount. All traumatized and devitalized tissue must be absorbed and replaced during the process of healing and forms a nidus for postoperative infection. Avoidance of excessive cautery, large fleshy pedicles and large areas of dead space will all contribute to an uncomplicated recovery.
3. Instruments and sutures. Gynecological surgeons have often and justifiably been criticized for the size of the instruments used. In this type of surgery as in any other, the smallest forceps or other instrument that will suffice should be chosen to avoid leaving large amounts of devitalized tissue in the suture.

Similarly suture material should not be chosen for its thickness. Suture material of any variety thicker than 0 (or 1 at the most) should not be used.

4. Hemostasis. This should be meticulous at all times. The judicious use of cautery, ligaclips, hemostatic materials and patience is essential. Pressure continued for a period of 4 minutes 'by the clock' will often stop troublesome oozing in the pelvis and do away with the necessity for clamps in inopportune places. Acute blood loss from a large vessel should always be dealt with immediately.
5. Drains. All areas (dead spaces) where more than 80–100 ml of fluid might accumulate postoperatively should be drained. Expensive suction type drains have no advantage over a properly placed corrugated or pencil drain.
6. Wound closure. There are almost as many methods of wound suturing as there are surgeons. Once again the basic principles: attention to detail avoiding tension and in particular meticulous hemostasis are important. The technique of mass closure using non-absorbable suture material is most appropriate for cancer surgery provided the above basics are observed.
7. Operative time. Individual operating time depends on many factors and will always differ for any given procedure. 'Clock watching' does not encourage good surgery. The golden rule for an individual surgeon is to perform the operation competently and safely without dawdling or wasting time because postoperative morbidity is directly related to operative time.
8. Catheterization. It is fashionable to insert suprapubic catheters after major gynecological operations. While these do have advantages over urethral catheters they are very expensive and should be used only where essential in developing countries. Urinary secretion should be carefully monitored and maintained at 40–50 ml per hour.
9. Where HIV status is not known preoperative measures such as wearing two pairs of gloves, the use of blunt needles, protective clothing, masks and vizors is important. Perhaps more important is careful technique to avoid injury to any of the operating team.

POSTOPERATIVE MANAGEMENT

The first 72 hours of this period are critical for optimum recovery and it should be decided pre- or intraoperatively whether the patient merits extra care. If intensive or high care units are not available special nursing and medical care should be arranged until the patient's condition is stable. The following aspects merit special attention.

1. General condition. Temperature readings should be taken every 4 hours together with other vital signs, pulse rate and blood pressure. Tissue perfusion and restlessness as well as untoward reactions to drugs must be monitored.
2. Cardiovascular system. In addition to pulse rate and blood pressure it is important to ensure that fluid overload does not occur and if central venous pressure monitoring is not available the lung bases and jugular venous pressure should be regularly checked.
3. Respiratory system. Clinical examination of the chest to ensure adequate ventilation, absence of atelectasis particularly at the lung bases and to exclude incipient infection or adult respiratory distress syndrome is important and should be routinely performed twice daily.
4. Urinary tract. The urinary output should be watched carefully and compared with the intake to ensure that a balance is maintained.

   The color of the urine gives early warning of oliguria, the specific gravity may be useful and while hematuria often is present for 24 hours after radical surgery, persistence or later occurrence is of significance.

   Oliguria frequently occurs and the cause should be determined early while easily correctable. Simple reasons such as inadequate fluid replacement or blocked catheter should be excluded before more elaborate investigations are instituted.
5. Gastrointestinal tract. A nasogastric tube is often required postoperatively. This should be removed as soon as possible. Removal is usually possible 24–48 hours after surgery when early propulsive bowel sounds are present but occasionally this must be delayed. Where doubt exists a gastric balance is useful. The nasogastric tube is clamped, the patient given 100 ml of fluid per mouth hourly for 8 hours and the residual measured at the end of this period. If the residual is less than 80 ml the tube can be removed.

   A definitive diagnosis must be made early if bowel complications occur. In particular the distinction must be made between an ileus and obstruction. This can usually be done on clinical grounds with the aid of an erect and supine abdominal X-ray. Judicious conservative management for the former and early surgery (often after a short period of conservative treatment) for the latter will often save the patient a long hospital stay.

In uncomplicated cases small amounts of oral fluid intake should be started earlier rather than later, often in the first 24 hours.

6. Peripheral vasculature. The prevention of thromboembolic complications is of paramount importance. Early ambulation in the first 24 postoperative hours, physiotherapy, the use of graduated pressure elastic stockings and the continuation of prophylactic heparin are key measures. High level clinical surveillance for early signs is necessary and the early use of Doppler ultrasound or venogram for confirmation is essential. In uncomplicated instances the prophylactic heparin can be discontinued as soon as the patient is fully mobile, usually on the fourth or fifth day.
7. Intravenous fluid intake. This should be monitored constantly to ensure adequate hydration and to exclude fluid overload, particularly in older people. If not discontinued after 48–72 hours, electrolytes, urea and creatinine should be monitored daily and early corrective action taken to correct any developing imbalance.
8. Wound sites. These should be inspected daily from the fifth postoperative day. Incipient wound infection is best treated early and in particular collections of fluid (blood or pus) should be drained as soon as evident. In uncomplicated cases sutures can be removed on the seventh day after operation.
9. Analgesia and anti-nauseant drugs. Whatever preparations and routes are used this often neglected aspect of postoperative care must be optimal.

   Epidural anesthesia and patient demand systems using opiates are excellent and should be used where available. Where not available, intramuscular analgesic injections supplemented by rectal non-steroidal anti-inflammatory suppositories given regularly every 4–6 hours are favored. Similarly, anti nauseant drugs must be given by intravenous or intramuscular injection whenever required.

DISCHARGE FROM HOSPITAL AND FOLLOW-UP

1. A full explanation of the operative procedure is required including:
   (a) The prognosis.
   (b) Additional treatment required and why.
   (c) Exactly which organs were removed and which conserved.
   (d) The effects on femininity and sexual function.
   (e) The effects on body image.
2. Appropriate hormone replacement therapy should be discussed and prescribed.

3. Arrangements should be made for follow-up and the importance of these visits explained.

CONCLUSIONS

The general principles of care before, during and after surgery have been described in detail. If these principles are adhered to benefits for the patient will be maximized, complications will occur less frequently, recovery will be more rapid and the duration of hospitalization reduced. Only attention to detail will achieve these aims.

9

Cancer of the vulva

C.M.C. Dehaeck

INTRODUCTION

Vulval cancer is uncommon and accounts for approximately 1–4% of all gynecological cancers, an incidence of 1.8 per 100 000. It is predominantly seen in postmenopausal and older women (mean age 65 years) and after the age of 70 years the incidence peaks at 20 per 100 000. In countries such as South Africa, where sexually transmitted diseases are common, the mean age of presentation is 59 compared with 65 years reported elsewhere. Women often present with this disease at a late stage especially in developing countries and this can pose a management problem. Although many types of malignancy can arise in the vulval area, for the purpose of the chapter the main focus will be on squamous invasive vulval cancer.

EPIDEMIOLOGY

This is covered in Chapter 1.

CLINICAL FEATURES AND DIAGNOSIS

The most common presenting complaint is a vulval ulcer or mass. Patients also present with pruritus, bleeding, discharge or less frequently with a metastatic groin mass. Even though this cancer is very easily detected at an early stage by the woman herself, it often is advanced by the time she seeks help. This is commonly the case in countries where transport and medical facilities are less than optimal. An additional explanation is that older women are often embarrassed and shy. On examination these lesions can take on any form from a flat white lesion to a large ulcerative crater. Attention should be given to any discolored area and warty lesion. These are often dismissed as condylomata acuminata and are locally destroyed without biopsy, which may delay diagnosis and treatment.

Diagnosis is made on histology from a punch biopsy, wedge biopsy or an excision biopsy if the lesion is small enough to be completely excised. Care must be taken to provide the pathologist with some surrounding normal skin and underlying connective tissue so that depth of invasion can be assessed.

STAGING

The International Federation of Gynecology and Obstetrics (FIGO) suggest a clinical staging based on the TNM classification taking into consideration the size of the local lesion, groin node involvement and metastases. Postsurgical staging is more accurate as involvement of the groin lymph nodes is missed on clinical examination in up to 30% of cases and overdiagnosed in 50%. Staging procedures include a clinical assessment, aspiration cytology of groin nodes if enlarged and a chest X-ray.

Refer also to Chapter 7.

PROGNOSIS

The overall 5 year survival rate for vulval cancer is quoted as 70% for all operable cases. This is dependent on:

1. Lymph node involvement. This is the most important prognosticator. Metastatic involvement of groin nodes decreases the 5 year survival rate to below 50% as opposed to the 90% when lymph nodes are not involved. Once pelvic nodes are involved the 5 year survival rate is only 15%.

   The presence of malignant groin nodes is related to the size of the tumor. In FIGO stage I (<2 cm in diameter) the incidence is 10–13%. This increases to 26% in FIGO stage II and to 64% in stage III.

   Metastases to the pelvic nodes are related to the size of the vulval tumor. If the tumor is less than 4 cm in diameter the incidence of pelvic node involvement is virtually zero as opposed to a larger tumor where it is 7%.

   The number of groin nodes involved is another important factor in survival. One microscopically involved lymph node regardless of the stage has a good prognosis while two or more positive nodes have a worse prognosis. Only 26% of the latter patients are disease free at 5 years.
2. Stage. The 5 year survival decreases with advancing stage from >90% in stage I to <10% in stage IV.

3. Differentiation. A well-differentiated tumor has a better prognosis than a poorly differentiated tumor.
4. Depth of invasion. Depth of invasion and its influence on nodal metastases mainly applies to stage I disease. Invasion of 1 mm and less poses no risk for nodal metastases. Between 1 mm and 3 mm invasion there is a 6–8% incidence of groin lymph node positivity and between 3 mm and 5 mm invasion the incidence is as high as 22–37%. The practical problem for the pathologist is measuring the depth of invasion and it is probably more accurate measuring the total thickness of the lesion. If the total thickness is less than 3 mm there is <2% of nodal metastases.
5. Surgical margin. Finally, a surgical excision margin of more than 10 mm in all diameters results in a low local recurrence rate.

TREATMENT

The corner stone of treatment is surgery.

The majority of FIGO stages I and II will be cured by surgery alone. Because most vulval cancers present at an advanced stage in developing countries other treatment modalities such as chemotherapy and radiotherapy may have to be used.

SURGERY

The standard surgery of *en bloc* radical vulvectomy and bilateral groin node dissection as described by Taussig and Way was associated with a high incidence of morbidity, as well as problems with body image and sexual function. The recent trend is towards less radical surgery and individualization of the treatment depending on the size and position of the tumor, depth of invasion and the age and performance status of the patient.

The flow charts (Figs 9.1 and 9.2) depict the suggested approach to this disease and are based on the above risk factors.

Definitions for flow charts

Superficial invasion	<1 mm depth of invasion and <2 cm in diameter.
Lateral lesion	One which does not encroach on midline structures.
Central lesion	Involves a midline structure or is too close to the midline to be cleared by a surgical margin of 1 cm.

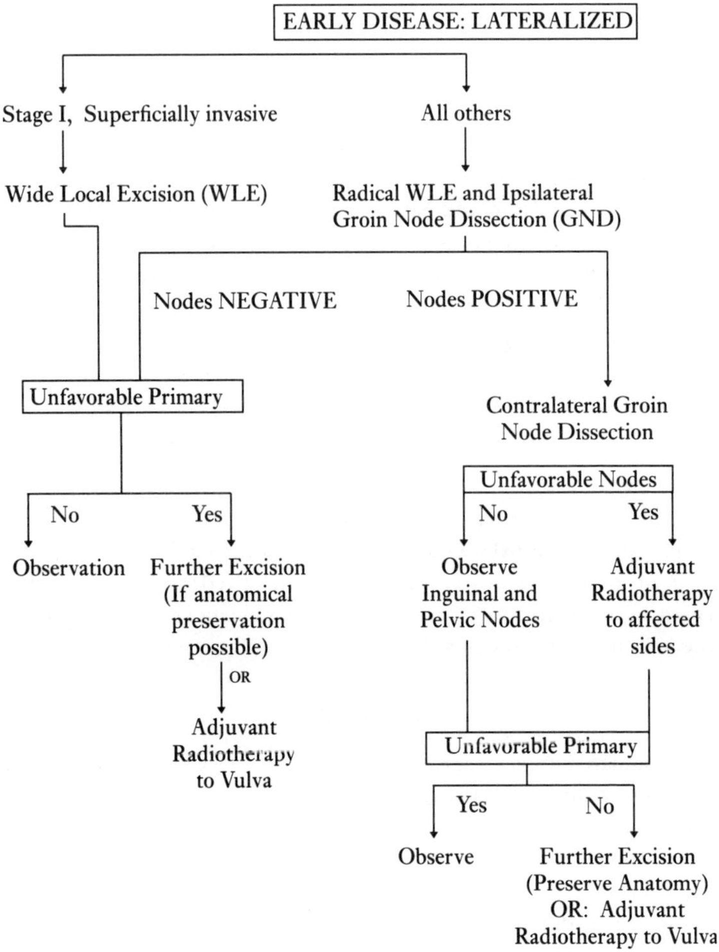

Fig. 9.1 Flow chart showing suggested approach to early lateralized disease of the vulva. (Redrawn from Thomas, G.M. *et al.* (1991) *Gynecologic Oncology* **42**: 9–21).

Early favorable disease	Clinically impalpable inguinal lymph nodes and radical excision of vulvar lesion can be accomplished without sphincter sacrifice.
Advanced disease	Clinically suspicious lymph nodes are present or radical excision of the vulvar tumor will require sphincter sacrifice.

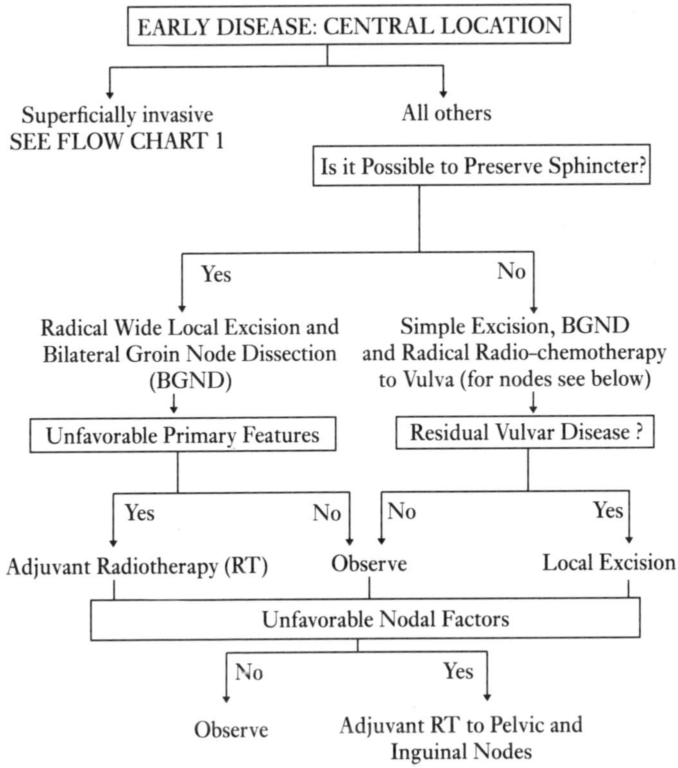

Fig. 9.2 Flow chart showing suggested approach to central location of early disease of the vulva. (Redrawn from Thomas, G.M. *et al.* (1991) *Gynecologic Oncology* **42**: 9–21).

Unfavorable nodal features	>2 nodes positive or single nodal metastasis >5 mm or extracapsular spread.
Unfavorable vulvar primary	Excision margins <1 cm free of tumor.
Wide local excision	Excision of lesion with 1 cm skin margin.
Radical wide local excision	Excision extends down to deep perineal fascia and clears the tumor by a margin of at least 1 cm in all directions.

STAGE I

In cases where there is less than 1 mm invasion or the full thickness of the lesion is less than 3 mm, wide local excision with margins of normal skin of more than 10 mm without groin node dissection is acceptable. All other cases need groin node dissection to assess:

- Nodal involvement
- Need for adjuvant therapy.

Individualization of treatment depends on whether a lesion is lateral or central. Lateral lesions have ipsilateral groin node dissection while all central lesions need bilateral groin node dissection.

The vulval lesion does not always require radical vulvectomy. Radical wide local excision can be performed provided the margin of normal skin excised is more than 10 mm.

Groin nodes can be removed via separate incisions. This decreases wound healing complications. Non-involved skin is not excised as spread to the nodes occurs by embolization.

STAGES II AND III

The treatment for all advanced stages is radical vulvectomy and bilateral groin node dissection. If two or more nodes are positive the patient needs further treatment in the form of pelvic radiotherapy or pelvic node dissection. The latter has a high operative and postoperative morbidity and therefore radiotherapy is the procedure of choice. However, where no radiotherapy is available it may be of value to proceed to pelvic node dissection.

Large lesions >4 cm or those involving the anal sphincter or urethra are better treated with initial concomitant radio/chemotherapy which will shrink the lesion. Thereafter local excision of residual tumor may be possible.

STAGE IV

Fortunately few patients present with advanced disease and distant metastases are rare. For the primary lesion, palliative surgery or radiotherapy may be considered while in isolated cases concomitant radio/chemotherapy can be offered. Alternatively management should be supportive in nature where radical treatment is inappropriate.

PREOPERATIVE MANAGEMENT

Radical vulval surgery is disfiguring and may lead to severe sexual dysfunction. It is therefore imperative that the patient and her partner are counseled.

COMPLICATIONS

Early complications

The most common complication of this surgery is that of groin wound infection, necrosis and breakdown. This occurs in up to 50% of cases and may require irrigation, sitz baths and allowing secondary wound granulation. Another important complication is pulmonary embolism and therefore it is important that the patient continues her thromboembolic prophylaxis until mobilization has been achieved.

Late complications

Leg edema has been reported in up to 60% of patients while posterior vaginal prolapse occurs in about 10% of patients. The most important late complication is that of sexual dysfunction and despite all precautions occurs in 80% of patients.

CHEMOTHERAPY AND RADIOTHERAPY

Where the primary lesion on the vulva is massive or would involve surgery which leaves the patient with non-functioning sphincters it may be advisable to treat initially with concomitant chemotherapy and radiotherapy. This leads to shrinkage of the primary tumor after which a local excision of the residual tumor is possible (Chapter 16). The regimen can also be used in elderly patients who may not be suitable for major surgery.

RECURRENT VULVAL CANCER

Recurrence may occur locally, in the groin nodes, the skin bridge between vulva and groin or in distant sites. Local recurrence can be treated either by surgical excision or alternatively, if the patient has not previously been subjected to radiotherapy, by local radiotherapy.

The survival of patients with recurrent vulval cancer is dependent on the site of the recurrence. In the vulval area adequate treatment with good long-term results is possible. However, groin node and distant recurrences are difficult to treat and have a poor prognosis.

OTHER VULVAL MALIGNANCIES

These comprise of a small percentage of the total. Melanoma, Bartholin gland carcinoma, basal cell carcinoma, verrucous carcinoma and sarcoma may occur. Melanoma and basal cell carcinoma are treated similarly to other sites. Bartholin gland carcinoma is managed identically to squamous cell carcinoma.

Verrucous carcinoma is a variant of squamous cell carcinoma and histologic diagnosis is difficult. Clinically it resembles a warty lesion and is associated with HPV infection. It is a slow growing and locally destructive type of lesion and treatment may pose a problem depending on the size and site of the tumor. Surgery is the treatment of choice. Spread to regional lymph nodes is rare and local excision is adequate. The response to radiotherapy is variable. It is not uncommonly seen in developing countries.

10

Cancer of the vagina

B. Bloch

Primary vaginal cancer is rare and only accounts for 1 to 2% of gynecological cancers. Metastatic tumors are more common than primary cancers and are mainly from the cervix, uterus, vulva or trophoblastic tumors.

PRIMARY TUMORS

Squamous cell carcinoma

The mean age of presentation is around 60 years of age and this is the commonest histologic type (95%).

The epidemiology is discussed in Chapter 1 but it is important to note that at least 30% of these patients have been previously treated for preinvasive or invasive cervical cancer and this emphasizes the importance of cytologic follow-up in this latter group of patients. For this reason it is important that these patients are followed-up cytologically. Additionally, 60% of patients with vaginal cancer have had a hysterectomy, making vaginal vault cytology important in subsequent examinations. The major presenting symptom is irregular postmenopausal sero sanguinous discharge or bleeding and the findings will depend on the stage and nature (ulcerative or exophytic) of the tumors. Diagnosis is confirmed by an adequate biopsy taken from the growing edge of the tumor.

Staging of these tumors is according to FIGO (Chapter 7). In developing countries 75–80% present with stage III or IV disease.

Treatment is mainly by radiotherapy (Chapter 17). Surgery and chemotherapy have very limited application. The overall 5 year survival is around 40%.

Other cell types

Adenocarcinoma makes up 6–7% of these tumors, tend to occur in younger women (40–50 years old) and included in this group are the

DES-induced tumors occurring in children and young women (15–20 years old). These and the rarer tumor types (melanoma, sarcomas and verrucous carcinomas) are treated similarly to squamous cell cancer. The exceptions are embryonal rhabdomyosarcoma (sarcoma botryoides) and germ cell tumors which respond exceptionally well to chemotherapy.

METASTATIC TUMORS

The diagnosis is made on clinical grounds and biopsy. Treatment is that of the primary neoplasm.

11

Cancer of the cervix

R.P. Soeters

INTRODUCTION

Cancer of the cervix is the most common female malignancy in developing countries. Unfortunately, a large proportion of patients present with advanced disease and are in a deplorable nutritional state. With the current social and economic trends it is not likely that there will be any change in the incidence of cancer of the cervix in developing countries. If anything, an increase of the incidence is expected possibly related to HIV-positive patients. Because of these circumstances, the limited access to sophisticated treatment modalities and the well-known lack of patient compliance, it is imperative that management of these patients should always be practically orientated.

SYMPTOMS

Although there are no symptoms characteristic of cancer of the cervix, vaginal discharge is found in 80–90% of patients. Abnormal bleeding, either pre- or postmenopausal, is another common presenting symptom. Postcoital bleeding, traditionally associated with cancer of the cervix, is a relatively uncommon complaint.

Patients with advanced disease, common in developing countries, may present with weight loss but above all with malodorous vaginal discharge due to a large tumor bulk infected by anerobic organisms. Other symptoms in advanced disease include urinary frequency and incontinence (vesicovaginal fistula), fecal incontinence (recto-vaginal fistula) and pelvic pain.

DIAGNOSIS

The place of Papanicolaou smears in the diagnosis of preinvasive lesions of the cervix is pre-eminent but unfortunately limited in the diagnosis of invasive cancer of the cervix. Because of the frequent presence of ulceration, infection and bleeding Papanicolaou smears render an unacceptably high false negative rate in patients with invasive cancer. When on clinical examination the cervix looks suspicious and abnormal, biopsies are indicated. A biopsy should be taken from the center of the tumor and another from the growing edge of the tumor. Bleeding caused by the biopsies can easily be controled with either silver nitrate or if more severe with an astringent like Monsel's solution. Both should be applied to the tumor only.

Conditions to be considered in the differential diagnosis of cancer of the cervix are chronic cervicitis, chancroid, tuberculosis, lymphogranuloma venereum, amoebiasis, schistosomiasis and syphilitic ulcers.

OTHER PHYSICAL FINDINGS

The majority of patients are normal on general physical examination. Occasionally in advanced disease a patient might have enlarged lymph nodes either in the supraclavicular or more rarely in the inguinal region.

A speculum examination is imperative in a patient who presents with abnormal vaginal bleeding. The local extent of the tumor should be recorded on inspection of the cervix. The speculum should after introduction into the vagina and inspection of the cervix be carefully rotated for 180° to inspect for vaginal metastasis or a coexistent vaginal primary lesion. Rarely a patient might present with a normal-looking cervix and one or more vaginal metastases. An endocervical tumor, the so-called barrel-shaped cervix, might also account for a normal-looking cervix.

STAGING

The FIGO staging classification is discussed in Chapter 7.

Accurate clinical staging in cancer of the cervix is essential and serves a number of purposes. First, a standard technique of assessing the extent of the disease is used. This serves to individualize treatment according to predesignated protocols. Staging can also be used to prognosticate for the individual patient. Second, it may be employed to compare stage distribution, treatment modalities and results of treatment between centers and within a particular center.

In order to make staging a purposeful exercise an understanding of the patterns of spread of cancer of the cervix is required (Table 11.1).

Table 11.1 Patterns of spread in cancer of the cervix

- = Direct invasion into cervical stroma, vagina, endometrium and parametrium
- = Lymphatic metastases
  - – Obturator fossa lymph node group
  - – Internal/external iliac lymph node groups
  - – Common iliac lymph node group
  - – Para-aortic lymph node chain
  - – Mediastinal lymph node chain
  - – Supraclavicular lymph nodes
- = Hematogenic metastases
  - – Liver
  - – Lung
- = Intraperitoneal metastases

Clinical staging

According to the FIGO guidelines, clinical staging may include examination (under anesthesia), cystoscopy, chest X-ray, intravenous pyelogram (IVP), proctoscopy and selected skeletal films where indicated. Unfortunately, none of these investigations carry a high accuracy rate and most have a low yield.

Examination of the patient does not always have to be carried out under anesthesia. Most of the patients in developing countries present at a late stage where involvement of the parametria is obvious. However, it might be unclear whether there is parametrial involvement due to cancer or whether parametrial thickening and/or nodularity is the result of previous or current pelvic inflammatory disease (PID). In these cases it is useful to prescribe a course of antibiotics followed a week later by an examination under anesthesia. Acute PID is managed similarly until WBC and ESR are normal when a treatment decision can be made.

Examination, whether or not under anesthesia, should always be carried out by at least two experienced gynecologists.

Cystoscopy has a low yield and at Groote Schuur Hospital this investigation is only carried out in stage IIa and higher. Even then, the pick-up rate is still very low. Furthermore, bladder involvement is sometimes difficult to assess but may be supported by urinary cytology. The significance of bullous edema is controversial but is not considered to signify bladder involvement.

Chest X-ray also has a low yield for metastases but may pick up unrelated abnormalities like tuberculosis.

The role of IVP has recently come under scrutiny and is rapidly being replaced by ultrasound examination of kidneys and ureters. IVP may be useful in an early lesion where a radical hysterectomy is indicated and where congenital abnormalities, such as an abnormal ureteric system, is difficult to diagnose on ultrasound examination.

Proctoscopy is only indicated where involvement of the rectal mucosa in suspected. Equally, limited skeletal films are only useful when bony metastases are suspected. Both these investigations are rarely indicated and should not be employed for routine staging purposes. Not included in the FIGO guidelines for clinical staging, but essential for the work-up and therefore management of patients with cancer of the cervix, are laboratory investigations such as hemoglobin, liver and renal function tests.

It should be emphasized that in general only investigations which might change the management of patients with cancer of the cervix are warranted. Investigations with limited clinical significance do not have a practical role to play in the management of the scores of patients which populate the oncologic service of any given hospital in the developing countries.

Surgical staging

The role of surgical staging is currently mainly investigational and has as yet not improved survival. Surgical staging has demonstrated that clinical stage underestimates the extent of disease, chiefly because of occult nodal metastases. The incidence of positive para-aortic nodes for stages I, II and III is approximately 10, 15 and 30%, respectively.

TREATMENT

The primary treatment of patients with cancer of the cervix can be subdivided into three categories:

1. Surgical treatment which is limited to patients with early disease, i.e. stages Ib and IIa.
2. Radiotherapy which can be used with certain restrictions in all stages.
3. Chemotherapy which plays a minor role at present.

Surgical treatment

The indications for a radical hysterectomy are limited to patients who have localized disease (stages Ia(ii), Ib and IIa), are in good physical condition, require maintenance of sexual function and who are not obese. The upper age limit is individualized and depends on the general condition of the patient.

The size of the tumor should play a role in management decisions as a large tumor is more difficult to excise and carries a high risk for lymph node metastasis. In general, surgery is not recommended for a lesion greater than 4 cm in its largest diameter.

Finally, the indications for surgery will depend on the available surgical skills and the accessibility of a radiotherapy unit. The extent of primary surgical treatment depends mainly on the stage of the tumor. In the earliest stage (stage Ia(i)) conization might be definitive treatment whereas in the later stages (stage Ib and IIa) radical hysterectomy and pelvic lymph node dissection is more appropriate.

Piver and Rutledge have classified the classes of hysterectomy according to the extent of the procedure and their indications:

1. Class I, also called extrafascial hysterectomy. The aim of this procedure is to remove all cervical tissue including the paracervical fascia.

   This procedure is indicated in stage Ia(i) disease and early stage Ia(ii) (i.e. between 1 and 3 mm stromal invasion) without endothelial lined space involvement. It might also be indicated in patients with adenocarcinoma *in situ*.
2. Class II is also referred to as the modified radical hysterectomy. Its aim is to remove the medial half of the cardinal and uterosacral ligaments and ligation of the uterine vessels just medial to the ureters. The upper one-third of the vagina is removed. This procedure is indicated for patients who present with late stage Ia(ii) (i.e. between 3 and 5 mm stromal invasion) without endothelial lined space involvement.
3. Class III (Meigs') differs from class II insofar as the uterine arteries are ligated lateral to the ureter at their origin to the internal iliac arteries. In addition to removal of more paravaginal tissue, a pelvic lymph node removal is routinely performed. Class III operations are reserved for patients with late stage Ia(ii) (i.e. invasion between 3 and 5 mm) in combination with endothelial lined space involvement and stages Ib and IIa.
4. Class IV is aimed at removal of all paraureteral and more paravaginal tissue together with excision of the superior vesical arteries and three-quarters of the vagina. This operation is mainly indicated in patients with a central recurrence after radiotherapy where preservation of the bladder is still possible.

5. Class V differs from class IV in that distal sections of the ureter and/or bladder are removed. Class V operation might be considered in patients with a central recurrence after radiotherapy with involvement of the bladder base.

Ovarian preservation is always recommended in young patients where the maintenance of ovarian and sexual function is important.

Ovarian suspension may be considered if an intraoperative assessment strongly suggests the possibility of postoperative radiotherapy. This procedure entails a dissection of the infundibulopelvic ligament beyond the intersection with the ureter and subsequent attachment of the ovary to the lateral abdominal wall in order to place the ovary outside the fields of external radiation. The ovaries can be marked during the procedure with radiopaque clips to assist the radiotherapist for easier location.

Finally, it should be emphasized that where a patient presents with advanced disease and radiotherapy is not available there is no indication for surgical treatment. Only palliative surgical treatment may be indicated.

The surgical treatment of microinvasive carcinoma is confusing and controversial because of the dispute surrounding definitions. The treatment must be seen as an exercise in balancing the risks of pelvic lymph node metastasis against the complication rate of extended surgical treatment.

The FIGO guidelines for the diagnosis of microinvasive carcinoma have been included in the FIGO staging system (Chapter 7). The Society of Gynecologic Oncologists (SGO), however, state that a microinvasive carcinoma is to be defined as 'a neoplastic lesion which invades the stroma to a depth of less than or equal to 3 mm in the absence of lymphatic or blood vascular involvement'.

Based on these two definitions and on the risk for lymph node metastasis, the extent of the operation can be determined (Table 11.2).

POSTOPERATIVE COMPLICATIONS

The risk of surgical complications after radical hysterectomy is relatively low and depends mainly on the experience of the surgeon. It is also determined by concomitant medical conditions such as chronic PID and previous pelvic surgery.

The most common complications after radical hysterectomy have been listed in Table 11.3. A well-known immediate complication after radical hysterectomy is urethral fistula but the incidence now is only

Table 11.2 Indication for treatment of patients with microinvasive carcinoma of the cervix

Treatment	*Indication*	*Risk for lymph node metastasis (%)*
Cone biopsy	Young patient <3 mm ELSI: negative	<0.1
Vaginal or abdominal hysterectomy	<3 mm ELSI: negative	<0.1
Abdominal hysterectomy and pelvic lymphadenectomy	>3 mm and <5 mm ELSI: negative	<5
Class II radical hysterectomy	>3 mm and <5 mm ELSI: positive	<5
Class III radical hysterectomy	>3 mm and <5 mm Anaplastic tumor >7 mm width	

ELSI: endothelial lined space involvement.

Table 11.3 Common complications after radical hysterectomy

Complication	*Incidence (%)*
– Urethral fistula	1–2
– Bladder dysfunction	4–5
– Lymphocyst formation	2–5

1–2%. This is a marked decrease compared with three decades ago when the incidence was 10–15%. The main reasons for this decrease are improved surgical technique and routine drainage of the retroperitoneal space.

Another troublesome complication is bladder dysfunction which is usually transitory and affects most patients. The etiology is probably a surgical disruption of the autonomic nerve supply crossing the cardinal ligament resulting in a decreased urge to void. Prevention of the subsequent overdistension of the bladder is best accomplished by using a suprapubic catheter for at least 7 days.

The most common chronic postoperative complication is lymphocyst formation which only require drainage if they cause symptoms such as pain or urinary tract obstruction.

Other complications are not significantly more common than those associated with other pelvic operations.

Radiotherapy

Radiation therapy is extensively discussed in Chapter 16 but must be considered in the light of limited facilities typically associated with developing countries.

Chemotherapy

The results of chemotherapy in patients with cancer of the cervix are as yet not favorable. An overview is given in Chapter 15.

SPECIAL MANAGEMENT PROBLEMS

Cancer of the cervix complicated by pregnancy

Pregnancy-associated cancer of the cervix presents a special management problem as the obstetric mandate to deliver a healthy baby can be jeopardized by the need to treat the tumor.

Patients with pregnancy-associated cancer of the cervix are diagnosed at an earlier stage than non-pregnant patients and have a better prognosis overall. The main probable reason for this phenomenon is that pregnant patients are more readily exposed to a healthcare system. The survival rates after stratifying for stage show that the associated pregnancy *per se* has no influence. The prognosis therefore depends mainly on the extent of the disease.

Treatment also depends on extent of disease but is also influenced by gestational age (GA).

In the patient with early stage disease, management should be as follows:

1. First trimester and early second trimester (<20 weeks GA): radical hysterectomy.
2. Late second trimester and third trimester (>20 weeks GA): if indicated and desired by the patient wait for fetal viability; classical cesarean section followed immediately by radical hysterectomy.
3. Postpartum: radical hysterectomy.

With late stage disease, management should be as follows:

1. First trimester: ignore the pregnancy. Commence external therapy and await spontaneous abortion induced by the radiotherapy. After the abortion, brachytherapy is commenced to allow for better dosimetry.
2. Early second trimester: hysterectomy followed by external radiotherapy and brachytherapy.

3. Late second trimester and third trimester: if indicated await fetal viability. Classical cesarian section followed by external radiotherapy and brachytherapy.
4. Postpartum: treat as in the non-pregnant state.

Vaginal delivery should be avoided because it might cause catastrophic hemorrhage and theoretically possible spread of cancer cells. Occasionally a patient presents in labor with cancer of the cervix and without the choice of a surgical option. The prognosis for these patients does not seem to be adversely affected by vaginal delivery.

Adenocarcinoma of the cervix

Adenocarcinoma has traditionally been considered as a special management problem. However, it seems that squamous and adenocarcinoma are prognostically comparable when stratified for stage. Adenocarcinoma of the cervix does not warrant adjustments to the protocol used with squamous carcinoma of the cervix.

Patients with adenocarcinoma tend to present later than patients with a squamous lesion. The main reason is that an adenocarcinoma tends to arise in the endocervix with less obvious signs and symptoms.

Cancer of the cervical stump

Cancer of the cervical stump is rare but poses relatively few problems. Presenting signs and symptoms, diagnosis and treatment are essentially identical to this disease with the uterine body *in situ*. Survival rates after either surgery or radiotherapy are also comparable.

Pelvic inflammatory disease

PID creates special problems particularly related to treatment and complications. PID might result in the small bowel becoming adherent in the pelvis, which could lead to serious bowel disturbance after excess radiotherapy exposure.

Surgery is usually the treatment of choice where PID is associated with early cervical cancer. Radiotherapy in these circumstances often carries unacceptably high complication rates which may be fatal.

Cervical hemorrhage

In developing countries the majority of patients present with advanced cancer of the cervix with an increased risk of serious bleeding from the tumor.

A number of treatment options are available:

1. Monsel's solution and vaginal packing with bed rest (usually 48 hours) while the pack is in place.
2. Radium insertion after debulking of the tumor.
3. If radiotherapy facilities are not available a surgical approach, i.e. ligation of both internal iliac arteries, is indicated.

Recurrent cervical cancer

Most recurrences occur after radiotherapy as this treatment modality is reserved for patients with advanced disease.

With recurrent disease after radiotherapy repeat irradiation is not possible because of severe complications and no realistic hope for cure. Surgery may be the best approach with a local recurrence but it is of the utmost importance that regional and distant spread are excluded. Pelvic exenteration may be appropriate but most patients with recurrent disease will be managed more conservatively.

AIDS AND CANCER OF THE CERVIX

Patients who test positive for the human immunodeficiency virus (HIV) are at increased risk for developing CIN and cancer of the cervix. This is exemplified by findings of a 14% and 22% CIN rate in HIV patients in Malawi and Zaire respectively. Cancer of the cervix has been recognized as an indicator disease for HIV-positive status. This has relevance for developing countries as the rate of HIV infection and subsequent acquired immune deficiency syndrome (AIDS) is high and shows an exponential increase. This trend is most likely a result of irresponsible sexual behavior and the high rate of sexually transmitted diseases with concomitant existence of genital ulcers. A compounding factor is that in Sub-Saharan Africa more females than males are now HIV-positive.

At Groote Schuur Hospital, Cape Town, all patients with cancer of the cervix are tested for HIV. If positive the CD4 count is used as a parameter to monitor disease progression. These patients are extensively counseled and further examined for other associated conditions such as tuberculosis.

Management of these patients should be individualized but treatment for cancer of the cervix should not be withheld in a patient who is HIV-positive.

In patients with full blown AIDS the choice for curative treatment of the cancer of the cervix is more difficult as life expectancy and quality of future life are impossible to assess. Management of these patients requires a multidisciplinary approach.

POST-TREATMENT SURVEILLANCE

The majority of recurrences occur within 2 years after treatment. Follow-up visits should include a 2 monthly examination for this period and thereafter should be scheduled 4–6 monthly for 3 years.

Physical examination should include palpation of inguinal and supraclavicular lymph nodes and abdominal examination for abnormalities. The external genitalia should be carefully inspected with special attention to the vulva, lower vagina and paraurethral areas. After inspection of vagina and cervix a cytologic smear should be taken. On pelvic examination (per vagina and per rectum) special attention should be paid to the parametria, the size of the uterus (to exclude a pyometria after radiotherapy), masses and the status of rectal mucosa.

Finally, a chest X-ray film should be arranged every 12 months for at least 5 years after diagnosis.

PROGNOSIS AND SURVIVAL

Stage at presentation is ultimately the most important determinant of survival. Apart from initial stage a number of prognostic factors have been said to affect survival (Table 11.4). These prognosticators signify an increased risk for lymph node metastases.

The influence of stage on the survival rate of patients with cancer of the cervix is unquestionable. In addition, the lower 5 year survival rate according to stage in developing countries compared with that of developed countries highlights the differences between these two socio-economic environments.

The lower survival rate in developing countries is probably a result of malnutrition and poor patient compliance causing treatment disruptions. Improvement of primary healthcare and education may eradicate these anomalies.

Table 11.4 Prognosticators (apart from stage) in carcinoma of the cervix

1. Grade of the primary tumor
2. Size of the primary tumor
3. Involvement of endothelial lined spaces

12

Cancer of the corpus uteri

R.P. Soeters

INTRODUCTION

Two main types of malignancy may arise from the corpus uteri:
A. Endometrial carcinoma.
B. Sarcoma of the uterus.

The emphasis in this chapter will be on endometrial cancer as this is by far the most common of the two cancers.

CANCER OF THE ENDOMETRIUM

Histology

Although the histologic classification of endometrial carcinoma has been discussed in Chapter 2 special attention should be given to the malignant potential of endometrial hyperplasia where several classifications exist. A recent classification and approximate malignant potential of the types of hyperplasia is shown in Table 12.1.

Signs and symptoms

The most important symptom in all age groups is abnormal bleeding and in view of the age distribution most patients present with postmenopausal bleeding. Education must ensure that patients recognize such bleeding as abnormal and seek medical advice. Other less common symptoms are persistent bloody discharge and lower abdominal pain. Only a minority of patients are asymptomatic and the diagnosis may then be made after an abnormal cytologic smear or as an incidental finding after hysterectomy for other indications.

Diagnosis and physical examination

Endometrial sampling should be done on every postmenopausal patient who presents with vaginal bleeding. Prior to sampling of the

Table 12.1 Approximate malignant potential of endometrial hyperplasia

Type of hyperplasia	*Malignant potential (%)*
Simple	1–5
Complex	25
Atypical	50–75

endometrium a hysteroscopy may be carried out to investigate the nature and extent of the problem.

The classical practice for endometrial sampling has in the past been by fractional curettage but this procedure has become less prevalent with the introduction of the FIGO surgical staging classification in 1988.

Endometrial sampling rendering a cytologic result for the diagnosis of endometrial carcinoma is accepted and can be done as an office procedure. Numerous devices, such as Endo-Pap, Gravelee Jetwasher and Pipelle are available, are equally effective and relatively inexpensive. The interpretation of endometrial samples is difficult and requires a great deal of experience. More so in the case of endometrial hyperplasia which is notoriously difficult to diagnose on a cytologic specimen. In such a case sampling for histologic purposes is mandatory for accurate diagnosis.

Diagnostic dilatation and curettage is the most commonly performed operative gynecological procedure, provides a histologic diagnosis and is considered the gold standard for the diagnosis of endometrial carcinoma.

Physical examination of a patient with endometrial carcinoma is frequently entirely normal. This should include palpation of supraclavicular and inguinal lymph nodes. Abdominal palpation might be difficult due to obesity.

A gynecological examination should include a careful inspection of the vaginal skin in the suburethral area which is a relatively common site for metastases. Bimanual rectovaginal examination assesses uterine size and mobility, state of the parametria and adnexa.

Preoperative metastatic work-up should include full blood count, liver and renal function tests and chest X-ray. Other investigations are only indicated when there is a clinical suspicion that metastases are present. These might include proctoscopy and/or sigmoidoscopy, cystoscopy and in exceptional cases a bone scan.

Staging and pathophysiologic behavior

The FIGO staging classification has been discussed in Chapter 7. The staging was changed in 1988 from a clinical staging to a surgical staging which is far more realistic and accurate. This is exemplified by the detection of extrauterine spread in 25–30% of patients with clinical stage I disease.

Prognosticators such as grade of the primary tumor and myometrial invasion are part of the surgical staging and like vessel invasion are related to nodal disease (Table 12.2). Extrauterine spread may be in continuity to adjacent structures like adnexa and further afield to the pelvic and abdominal cavity. Lymphatic spread occurs to the pelvic and para-aortic lymph nodes and rarely in retrograde fashion to the suburethral area. In cases where pelvic nodes are involved more than 30% also have para-aortic lymph node metastases.

Hematogenous metastases are rare but are usually pulmonary.

Treatment

The mainstay of treatment for endometrial carcinoma is an extrafascial total abdominal hysterectomy and bilateral salpingo-oophorectomy (TAH-BSO).

The role of preoperative radiotherapy has become controversial with the introduction of the new (FIGO) staging system. Preoperative radiotherapy will severely affect the surgicopathologic staging.

Table 12.2 Risk factors and frequency of nodal metastases

Risk factor	*Pelvic (%)*	*Para-aortic (%)*
Grade		
well	3	2
moderate	9	5
poor	18	11
Myometrial invasion		
endometrium	1	1
superficial	5	3
middle	6	1
deep	25	17
Vessel invasion		
negative	7	9
positive	27	19

Creasman *et al.* (1987) *Cancer* **60**:2035–2041.

For all stages, except where widespread endometrial carcinoma is diagnosed preoperatively, a TAH-BSO is indicated. The operative technique for the TAH-BSO does not vary appreciably from that for a benign indication. The laparotomy is best performed through a lower midline abdominal incision to achieve adequate exposure of the abdominal cavity. After entering the abdomen washings are taken from the pelvis, paracolic gutters, and subdiaphragmatic area. The fluid is withdrawn and mixed with equal amounts of 50% alcohol for cytologic investigation. Thereafter a thorough laparotomy is performed followed by the TAH-BSO. Pelvic and para-aortic lymphadenectomy are indicated where high risk factors (grade, myometrial invasion, vessel invasion, cervical and adnexal involvement) are present (Table 12.2). A frozen section facility should be available to assess the presence of these high risk factors. An alternative would be an intraoperative macroscopic assessment of myometrial invasion immediately after the uterus is removed and bisected. Furthermore, gross involvement of extrauterine organs may be assessed to determine whether the patient is at risk for pelvic and para-aortic lymph node involvement. It should be stressed that indications for node sampling are only applicable when a radiotherapy unit is available.

Postoperative pelvic radiotherapy is aimed at sterilization of unsuspected often microscopic pelvic lymph node and vaginal metastases and is only indicated for selected high risk patients (Table 12.2).

Once the cancer has spread beyond the pelvis into the abdominal cavity there is no indication for postoperative radiotherapy and in such cases palliative treatment is indicated (Table 12.2).

The efficacy of current chemotherapy regimens in endometrial carcinoma is low and is still in an experimental stage (Chapter 15).

Survival

The 5 year survival of patients with endometrial carcinoma is essentially dependent on stage (Fig. 12.1). The impact of the change from clinical staging to surgical staging appears to be significant (Fig. 12.1).

There is not a great deal of difference between survival in developing countries and those of developed countries (Fig. 12.1). Other prognostic factors such as grade and vessel invasion also affect the survival rate.

The prognostic influence of peritoneal cytology is more controversial. There is evidence that positive peritoneal cytology alone does not

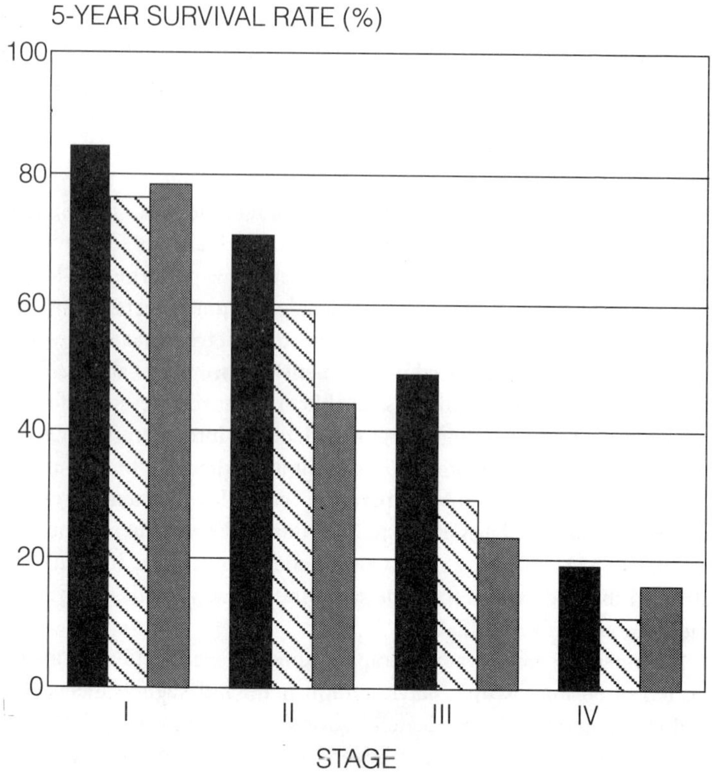

Fig. 12.1 Five year survival according to surgical (■), clinical (□) stage and in Groote Schuur Hospital (□). (Source: 21st Annual Report on Gynecological Cancer.)

influence the survival rate, but in combination with spread outside the uterus positivity has a significant adverse effect on survival.

Special management problems

1. Uterine serous papillary carcinoma (USPC). This is a rare but highly malignant adenocarcinoma of the endometrium which typically behaves like its ovarian counterpart. It is not uncommon for patients to present with gross ascites. The tumor has a propensity for intra-abdominal spread and the omentum is often involved. Treatment is similar to that of epithelial ovarian tumors and adjuvant chemotherapy should be platinum based. The prognosis is determined by stage of the tumor and is generally unfavorable.

2. Synchronous primary tumors of endometrium and ovary. This is a well-recognized albeit uncommon entity. The histologic features of both tumors are almost without exception those of an endometrioid adenocarcinoma. Each of these neoplasms should be treated as an isolated primary based on separate risk factors. The prognosis is generally favorable.
3. Recurrent disease. Treatment failures in patients with endometrial carcinoma will be detected in 70–75% within 2 years and in 10–20% after 5 years. In 50% of these patients only a local recurrence is found while in 30% a distant recurrence manifests. The remaining 20% have both a local as well as a distant recurrence. The single most common recurrence site is either the proximal or distal vagina. Depending on the number of recurrent foci, site of metastases and primary treatment the patient may be managed with surgery, radiotherapy, hormones or combination treatment. High dose medroxyprogesterone acetate will benefit approximately 40% of patients but for a limited period of 12–24 months.

UTERINE SARCOMAS

Uterine sarcomas are malignant tumors arising from either the myometrium (leiomyosarcoma) or the endometrium (others). These tumors are uncommon and account for under 5% of all uterine malignancies.

The age group commonly affected is 50 years or older. The most frequent presenting complaint is vaginal bleeding. On examination a pelvic mass may be found and occasionally a polypoid mass can be seen protruding from the cervix.

The histologic detail is found in Chapter 2 and the staging classification is the same as for endometrial carcinoma. The metastatic work-up for uterine sarcoma is also similar to that of endometrial carcinoma. These tumors often show locoregional spread but have a greater propensity for hematogenous spread with pulmonary metastases than endometrial cancer.

The cornerstone of the treatment for all uterine sarcomas is surgical, i.e. TAH-BSO. Intrapelvic disease is frequently encountered and occasionally upper abdominal spread may be found. Postoperative radiotherapy may be part of the treatment, although ultimate survival is not influenced.

The malignant behavior of uterine sarcomas is more aggressive than that of endometrial carcinoma and the 5 year survival rate in stage I is approximately 50%. In the case of extrauterine spread the 5 year survival rate is 20%.

A number of chemotherapeutic agents have been tested in patients with uterine sarcomas and the most active agents are adriamycin and cisplatinum. The survival rate is, however, not affected by adjuvant chemotherapy, with a minimal effect on disease-free interval.

13

Cancer of the ovary

E.W.W. Sonnendecker

EPIDEMIOLOGY

Carcinoma of the ovary is commoner in developed countries, such as Europe and the USA, than in the Third World. On the basis of the SEER (Surveillance, epidemiology and end result) data gathered in the USA, about 1.4% or 1 of every 70 newborn girls will develop cancer of the ovary at some time during their lives. However, it has been shown that in the Black population in South Africa the relative low frequency of epithelial tumors no longer applies.

Epithelial tumors account for 85–90% of the primary malignant tumors. They are uncommon before 35 years of age but the incidence increases rapidly with age thereafter to a peak in the 50–70-year-old age group.

Classification of ovarian tumors

Refer also to Chapter 2.

Table 13.1 sets out the histologic subtypes of ovarian tumors encountered at the laboratories associated with the University of the Witwatersrand and confirms that epithelial tumors are by far the most frequently encountered. Consequently this chapter will essentially address epithelial cancer whereafter the other subtypes will be briefly considered.

ETIOLOGY OF EPITHELIAL CANCERS

Refer also to Chapter 1.

Clinical presentation

SYMPTOMS

Ovarian carcinoma is insidious in onset, may be asymptomatic and does not present with specific symptoms. As the tumor enlarges, its

Table 13.1 WHO histologic classification of ovarian cancers

Histogenetic cell type	*Johannesburg Hospital*		*Southern Transvaal*	
	No	*%*	*No*	*%*
Common epithelial	112	92.6	615	53.4
Sex cord/stromal	2	1.6	95	8.2
Germ Cell	7	5.8	334	29.0
Lipid	–	–	–	–
Gonadoblastoma	–	–	–	–
Lymphoma	–	–	2	0.2
Unclassified	–	–	27	2.3
Secondary	–	–	58	5.0
Residual tumors*	–	–	22	1.9
Total	121	100	1153	100

*Ovaries not received for histopathology, but tumor elsewhere had the characteristics of a metastatic deposit from a primary ovarian tumor.
The series at the Johannesburg Hospital reported by Sonnendecker (1988) consisted of White patients and includes only primary malignant tumors. Ricklan's 1992 analysis pertains to Black patients in the Southern Transvaal and includes benign, Borderline and malignant tumors.

weight and the space it occupies cause urinary frequency or urgency, constipation, a sense of heaviness in the pelvis, occasional sharp twinges or dyspareunia. With growth beyond 12–15 cm in diameter or ascites, abdominal enlargement begins. Other frequent symptoms are non-specific gastrointestinal manifestations in 50% of patients which include vague abdominal discomfort, flatulence, gastrointestinal unrest, feeling of fullness after a light meal, slight loss of appetite and other mild digestive disturbances.

Abnormal uterine bleeding is a relatively infrequent symptom in women with ovarian epithelial malignancy.

Ovarian carcinoma may uncommonly present as a surgical emergency because of torsion, rupture or intra-abdominal hemorrhage.

PHYSICAL FINDINGS

In 40–75% of patients there is a palpable abdominal mass, 20–30% have clinically detectable ascites and 10% a pleural effusion. Only 1–2% of cases will have a negative examination. The most common mistaken preoperative diagnosis is uterine fibroids. The bimanual rectovaginal palpation of the pelvic organs is essential. The presence of cul de sac nodularity is an indication of malignancy and should not be treated as endometriosis without visual confirmation. If an adnexal or pelvic mass is solid, fixed, irregular, nodular, bilateral and large (10 cm), it is most likely to be malignant. Paradoxically, the extremely large ovarian tumors are usually benign mucinous cystadenomas. A large omental metastasis is often ballotable and has a solid, irregular feel.

METASTATIC SPREAD

The pelvic peritoneum and other pelvic organs become involved by direct spread. The peritoneal fluid, flowing to lymphatic channels on the undersurface of the diaphragm, carries malignant cells to the omentum, to the peritoneal surfaces of the small and large bowel and liver and to the parietal peritoneal surfaces throughout the abdominal cavity and on the surface of the diaphragm. Metastases on the undersurface of the diaphragm may be found in up to 44% of what otherwise seem to be Stage I–II disease. Hematogenous spread usually occurs late, mainly to the liver and the lung. Metastases to bone and brain are rare.

STAGING OF OVARIAN CANCER

Refer to Chapter 7.

DIAGNOSIS

The diagnosis of ovarian carcinoma ultimately depends on operative intervention. It is customary to utilize extensive preoperative evaluation to exclude other causes of a pelvic mass. However, operative findings correlate poorly with comprehensive preoperative special investigations. It is practical to limit routine work-up to the following: serum CA-125, lactate dehydrogenase (LDH) and liver function tests, ultrasonography of the pelvis and abdomen, chest X-Ray, stool occult blood and in selective cases barium enema.

If pleural fluid is present, it is evaluated cytologically. Ascites, however, is only examined cytologically if no pelvic mass is palpated. Fine needle biopsy is not recommended.

Numerous studies have demonstrated the value of preoperative serum CA-125 measurements in identifying patients with pelvic malignancy. Elevated CA-125 values can also be associated with pregnancy, endometriosis, adenomyosis, benign ovarian tumors and inflammatory conditions of the peritoneum etc. Mucinous carcinomas are less likely to cause elevated CA-125 values. Carcinoembryonic antigen (CEA) is abnormal most often in mucinous cystadenoma.

SURGICAL THERAPY

General principles

Surgery is the cornerstone of both the diagnosis and treatment of ovarian cancer. A vertical incision is mandatory for an adequate exploration of the upper abdomen. Before any manipulation of the tumor, a sample of ascitic fluid or of peritoneal saline washings must be taken for cytology. The whole abdomen must be inspected carefully with special attention being given to the omentum, the subdiaphragmatic areas, anterior abdominal wall, paracolic gutters, surface of the large and small bowel and the pelvic organs. If accessible the pelvic and para-aortic nodes are palpated. Suspicious peritoneal surfaces should be biopsied; routinely, biopsies should be obtained from the anterior, parietal, paracolic gutters and pelvic peritoneum to exclude occult disease. We regard thorough preoperative bowel preparation as mandatory as 30% of patients with a so-called normal barium meal required a bowel resection and only 61% of patients with radiologic evidence of bowel involvement needed a bowel resection.

The basic principle of surgical therapy for ovarian carcinoma is to remove the primary lesion and all metastases without putting the patient's life in immediate jeopardy. The standard therapeutic surgery for ovarian cancer is total abdominal hysterectomy with bilateral salpingo-oophorectomy (BSO) and omentectomy. Palpable nodes should be excised for study in all but the most advanced cases.

Tumor debulking or cytoreductive surgery

The only variables that are independently significant to survival are stage, grade, histologic type and the amount of tumor remaining after operation. Survival was uniformly poor if the diameter of the largest residual tumor mass exceeded 1.5 cm, irrespective of the total volume of tumor before resection. While survival was significantly related to the size of the largest residual mass, there was no difference in survival among patients with masses greater than 1.5 cm in diameter. The most aggressive surgery should be reserved for those cases in which all or nearly all of the gross tumor can be excised. It is this group of patients who stand to gain most by extending the surgical procedure to include resection of adjacent viscera. Most commonly the latter includes the sigmoid colon and rectum (anterior resection). If the pelvic tumor mass is large or densely adherent to the pelvic side wall and the colon, it is usually easier to enter the retroperitoneal space at the pelvic brim in order to ligate the ovarian vessels, dissect the ureter from the pelvic peritoneum and mobilize the tumor and the pouch of Douglas. The uterus is then usually removed retrograde in continuity with the tumor mass and the rectum mobilized from the hollow of the sacrum. The mass can sometimes be freed from the bladder and rectum by peeling the tumor-bearing visceral peritoneum off the underlying organ but frequently resection of part of the bladder or anterior resection is necessary.

In order to achieve optimal cytoreduction the surgery should be performed by surgeons who have been trained in gynecological oncology surgery.

Thus patients with suspected ovarian cancer should be referred to a gynecological oncology center before surgery.

Conservative surgery

The minimal treatment for ovarian carcinoma is unilateral salpingo-oophorectomy (USO) which is justifiable in a woman younger than 35 years of age whose family is not complete and who has a unilateral tumor which fulfils the criteria summarized in Table 13.2. Partial omentectomy and peritoneal cytology are also part of the operative procedure. Biopsy of the healthy-looking contralateral ovary is not justifiable because of the risk of mechanical infertility or even ovarian failure. If the tumor is found to be poorly differentiated or if the washings are positive, a second operation to clear the pelvis may be advizable. If an ovarian endometrioid carcinoma is diagnosed histologically, hysteroscopy and endometrial curettage at a later date will exclude a co-existent tumor in the endometrial cavity.

Table 13.2 Criteria for conservative surgical therapy (unilateral salpingo oophorectomy) in ovarian carcinoma

1. Stage Ia
   a) No ascites
   b) No dense adhesions
   c) No surface excrescences
   d) Unruptured
   e) Unilateral, confined neoplasm
2. Adequate surgical-pathologic evaluation
   a) Borderline or Grade I histology
   b) Negative peritoneal washings
   c) Negative omentum
   d) Negative evaluation of opposite ovary
   e) Negative endometrial biopsy

It is recommended in patients whose fertility has been preserved, that the residual adnexum and uterus be removed on completion of childbearing because the long-term risk for ovarian carcinoma may be significantly higher than that for women in general.

Intervention debulking surgery

Even with experienced surgeons patients will have irresectable ovarian carcinoma. In this situation, at least an entire involved ovary should be excised for definitive diagnosis. Thereafter two to four courses of cytoreductive chemotherapy are given and a second laparotomy may be performed in those women who respond.

Second-look surgery

The term second-look applies specifically to a laparotomy undertaken after 6–12 courses of chemotherapy to determine whether the patient with a complete clinical response is surgically and pathologically free of disease. In the absence of gross tumor, the second-look laparotomy involves multiple biopsies and cytologies in a concerted effort to detect any residual disease.

Such an operation is more specific and sensitive than any other method of measuring residual tumor but unfortunately a negative second-look laparotomy is not equivalent to a cure. The reported relapse rate for this group of patients is 25–50%. The fact that neither the surgical resection of residual tumor nor the opportunity to change the treatment based on the findings have any proven effect on the patient's long-term survival are other cogent arguments against second-look surgery.

It must thus be concluded that until an effective consolidation therapy becomes available, the second-look procedure should be limited to clinical trials.

CHEMOTHERAPY

Refer to Chapter 15.

SALVAGE THERAPY

As already indicated, there is no proven effective salvage regimen for patients with a positive second-look and secondary surgery for recurrent disease following definitive primary cytoreductive surgery and adequate cisplatin-based chemotherapy remains problematic and unhelpful. High dose progestin or tamoxifen may be used in selected patients where hormone receptors have been measured. The role of ifosfamide and taxol is still to be determined.

TREATMENT OF BORDERLINE TUMORS

The majority of ovarian neoplasms in the Borderline malignant category occur in women of reproductive age and are stage I at the time of diagnosis. The latter cases are adequately managed by unilateral salpingo-oophorectomy. For serous tumors, the opposite ovary should be carefully evaluated for evidence of bilateralism. If the patient is not desirous of fertility, a hysterectomy with bilateral adnexectomy and omentectomy is recommended. Where tumors are more advanced than stage I, the cornerstone of therapy is pelvic clearance. The role of postoperative chemotherapy or radiation therapy in such cases is unresolved.

PSEUDOMYXOMA PERITONEI

This term is generally used to refer to a more or less chronic state of viscid, mucinous 'ascites' which cannot be drained by paracentesis, thus requiring repeated laparotomy for removal of the material and/or encysted masses because of discomfort, distention or bowel obstruction. Pseudomyxoma peritonei is nearly always associated with a ruptured benign or malignant but especially Borderline mucinous tumor of the ovary or appendix, although the lesion may be microscopic in dimension. Treatment consists of hysterectomy, bilateral salpingo-oophorectomy, removal of the mucin, excision of the involved peritoneum along with appendicectomy. Postoperative systemic chemotherapy utilizing the CAP regimen, has been used and repeated laparotomy with re-evacuation of mucin, resection of encysted masses and relief of bowel obstruction, is often necessary.

RESULTS OF TREATMENT

The results of treatment of epithelial ovarian cancer vary considerably depending on histologic type, stage and grade, volume of disease left at completion of the primary surgical procedure and chemotherapy employed. The 4 year survival of patients with advanced disease (stages III and IV) treated at the Johannesburg Hospital in 1977 when surgical resection was less aggressive and chemotherapy consisted either of phenylalanine mustard alone or a combination of cyclophosphamide, methotrexate and 5-fluorouracil was only 4.4%. In 1987 the figure had improved to 42% following utilization of maximal surgical effort and cisplatin-based combination chemotherapy.

The 5 year survival rates for invasive epithelial ovarian cancer ranges from 60 to 70% in stage I disease to 10% in stages III–IV. Since the majority (approximately 75%) of patients present with advanced disease, the overall 5 year survival in the UK is only 23%.

In the case of Borderline epithelial tumors, the 5 year prognosis is good but the death rate continues to rise slowly thereafter.

PRIMARY PAPILLARY PERITONEAL NEOPLASMS (PPPN)

Normal-sized ovary carcinoma syndrome is a term which defines and encompasses various malignant conditions, either arising from the peritoneum or metastasizing to it, similar to widespread or localized tumors seen in epithelial ovarian cancer. Conditions which may express themselves clinically as normal-sized ovary (maximum diameter of 4 cm) carcinoma syndrome include:

1. Primary peritoneal papillary serous carcinoma (PPPSC).
2. Various forms of peritoneal mesothelioma.
3. Extra-ovarian epithelial tumors or mesenchymal neoplasms.
4. Metastatic tumors of the peritoneum.

PPPSC is the most common entity contributing to this syndrome. In most cases, the clinical presentation of this entity does not differ from that in the advanced stages of epithelial ovarian cancer nor from the presentation in other conditions causing normal-sized ovarian carcinoma syndrome, including widespread metastatic tumors of the peritoneum arising from the breast, thyroid, gastrointestinal tract, endometrium or pancreas.

Treatment of PPPSC is surgical, namely total abdominal hysterectomy with BSO and omentectomy followed by cisplatin-based chemotherapy regimens. CA-125 has been found useful in monitoring the course of the disease.

METASTATIC TUMORS OF THE OVARY

Approximately three-fourths of patients who have cancer metastatic to the ovaries will have the primary originating in the gastrointestinal tract, breast or uterus.

The relative incidence of metastatic ovarian cancer is quite difficult to establish accurately and figures vary greatly from 10 to 30%.

The most important means of spread of cancer from other sites to the ovary is via the rich network of intra-ovarian and extra-ovarian lymphatics, whose collecting trunks extend upward with the utero-ovarian vessels to the lumbar aortic and lateral caval nodes at the lower poles of the kidneys. Apart from lymphatic metastasis other routes include direct extension, dissemination through peritoneal fluid, metastasis through the lumen of the fallopian tube, hematogenous metastasis and iatrogenic via needle biopsies and paracentesis.

The treatment of choice for metastatic ovarian cancer is bilateral salpingo-oophorectomy, hysterectomy and omentectomy. Additionally, debulking of intra-abdominal tumor may be helpful in reducing the tumor mass before chemotherapy. The efficacy of chemotherapy for these patients is low but vigorous treatment of selected patients is probably worthwhile. The overall survival at 5 years was 12% and at 10 years was 7.5%.

NON-EPITHELIAL TUMORS

Malignant sex cord/stromal and germ cell tumors form a significant minority of ovarian malignancies in Southern Africa. As the behaviour and treatment of malignant germ cell and sex cord/stromal tumors differ from the epithelial variety, these groups are considered below.

Malignant germ cell tumors

The younger a patient is, the more common is the diagnosis of a germ cell tumor and the greater the likelihood that it is malignant. Approximately 60% of ovarian tumors in patients under 20 years of age are germ cell tumors and a quarter of these are malignant in girls younger than 15 years of age. In girls less than 10 years old, 84% of germ cell tumors are malignant whereas in adults the average figure is 5%.

Germ cell tumors are basically divided into three groups: those that are considered to arise from the undifferentiated gonadal cell, those arising from embryonic elements and those arising from non-embryonic components. In this chapter, only the common varieties will be discussed.

DYSGERMINOMA

Dysgerminoma forms 20–40% of malignant germ cell tumors. The presentation in over half the patients is non-specific but acute or chronic pain is commonly present. Children may have isosexual precocious puberty and menstrual disturbances may be associated with human chorionic gonadotrophin (HCG) production by isolated syncytiotrophoblastic cells within the tumor. Patients generally complain of abdominal distention or a lump in the abdomen and because the small pelvis of the child cannot contain masses of significant size, the tumor can be easily felt in patients who are not yet in their teens.

Lactate acid dehydrogenase (LDH), alpha-fetoprotein, HCG and CA-125 may be elevated and in many cases can serve as tumor markers. Because of the short half-life of some of these tumor markers, it is important to take a sample preoperatively or as soon after operation as possible.

The initial treatment approach for a patient suspected of having a malignant germ cell tumor (including dysgerminoma) is surgery for diagnosis, appropriate staging and therapy. Dysgerminoma is the only germ cell tumor with a high incidence of bilaterality (10–15%). The type of primary operative procedure depends on the surgical findings. In early stage unilateral disease, ipsilateral salpingo-oophorectomy, peritoneal cytologic specimens and random biopsies from the omentum, abdominal peritoneum, pelvic peritoneum and retroperitoneal nodes are indicated. Should the contralateral ovary appear abnormal or enlarged, a biopsy or ovarian cystectomy should be performed. If frozen section analysis reveals malignant disease or a dysgenetic gonad then bilateral salpingo-oophorectomy is indicated unless the disease is microscopic. The uterus should be preserved with possible view to assisted reproduction. If advanced disease is encountered, the principles applicable to cytoreductive surgery in advanced epithelial ovarian cancer should be followed.

The most important difference of dysgerminoma and other relatively common germ cell malignancies is their exquisite sensitivity to both chemo- and radiotherapy. It had thus in the past been standard therapy for the young patient with stage I disease to have unilateral salpingo-oophorectomy and either no further treatment or radiotherapy to the pelvis with the unaffected ovary shielded. Despite the latter, infertility may result following radiotherapy. This has changed with the advent of effective chemotherapy and an additional cogent reason for utilizing adjuvant chemotherapy rather than radiotherapy is the fact that 24% of dysgerminomas are mixed germ cell tumors which are not radiosensitive.

Second-look laparotomy in these patients is limited to those patients with advanced disease and known residual disease with initially negative serum tumor markers.

ENDODERMAL SINUS (YOLK SAC) TUMORS

The clinical features of the second most common ovarian malignant germ cell tumor are similar to those of dysgerminoma except that it is an extremely rapidly growing tumor which is more likely to present as an acute abdomen due to rupture following necrosis and hemorrhage. Symptoms occasionally mimic appendicitis. Moreover, it constantly secretes alpha-fetoprotein which is important in the monitoring of treatment. As many as 71% are stage I and involvement of the contralateral ovary does not occur in the absence of peritoneal spread. Surgical management is as for dysgerminoma. Surgery alone is ineffective; adjuvant chemotherapy with cisplatinum-containing regimens is mandatory.

TERATOMAS

Two types of malignancy occur in teratomas: malignant change in mature teratomas, which consists of malignant transformation of adult tissue and immature teratomas which are inherently malignant in their behavior. The most common malignancy in mature teratomas is a squamous carcinoma which occurs in about 1% of dermoid tumors. The prognosis is good if the squamous carcinoma is found incidentally as a small focus in an intact cyst. Where there has been rupture of the cyst or the tumor has penetrated the capsule, the prognosis is poor despite treatment.

Immature teratomas contain tissue from all three germinal layers. Seldom bilateral, they are often found to have extensive peritoneal metastases. Most patients present with pain. A major problem in the follow-up of these patients, who are managed as outlined for dysgerminoma and endodermal sinus tumors, is the irregular secretion of tumor markers. Disappearance of tumor markers does not guarantee, in these tumors, that complete remission has been obtained. Thus, in patients with more than stage I disease, and in patients with grade II or III tumor, a second-look operation is indicated at which as complete an excision of all suspicious areas as possible is performed.

EMBRYONAL CARCINOMA

Pure embryonal carcinoma is rare, accounting for no more than 5% of malignant ovarian germ cell tumors. The patient age range is 4–28 years (median 14 years) and with surgery and modern combination chemotherapy, a cure rate of 80% is expected.

MIXED (COMBINATION) GERM CELL TUMORS

Dysgerminoma and endodermal sinus tumor are the most common combination but other mixtures do occur. The choice of chemotherapy (following surgery) is tailored according to the mix of tumors present.

Mixed germ cell and sex cord/stromal tumors

This category contains large numbers of germ cells resembling mixtures of dysgerminoma cells and neoplastic gonadal stromal cells. The only significant tumor is the gonadoblastoma which is the commonest neoplasm arising in dysgenetic gonads and arises almost exclusively in them. Treatment is by combination chemotherapy.

Sex cord/stromal tumors

These tumors which are derived from the sex cords or mesenchyme of the embryonic gonad were previously referred to as gonadal stromal tumors. Many sex cord stromal tumors secrete sex steroids.

GRANULOSA CELL TUMORS: ADULT TYPE

Since the delineation of the juvenile granulosa cell tumor, it has become necessary to refer to the conventional form of this neoplasm as the 'adult type of granulosa cell tumor' which accounts for approximately 75% of sex cord/stromal tumors. One-third develop in women of reproductive age, the bulk of the remainder occurring in patients who have passed the menopause. Granulosa cell tumors which pursue a malignant course do so in a leisurely and indolent manner, with one-third of recurrences presenting more than 5 years after initial treatment. Recurrences can develop after as long a period as 25 years.

The surgical treatment is the same as for epithelial tumors.

A variant of granulosa cell tumor that tends to occur before puberty, but not exclusively in that age group, is the juvenile variety which has distinct histopathologic features.

SERTOLI AND SERTOLI-LEYDIG TUMORS

Previously called arrhenoblastomas or androblastomas, these sex cord/stromal tumors arise from cells exhibiting a testicular differentiation and may recapitulate stages in the development of the testis.

Approximately 10% of pure Sertoli cell tumors behave in a malignant fashion. Surgery as for granulosa cell tumors is the treatment of choice and chemotherapy may be used for metastatic or recurrent disease.

Miscellaneous mesenchymal tumors

Ovarian mesenchymal neoplasms are uncommon.

Malignant mixed Müllerian tumors (MMMT) (now called carcinosarcomas)

High grade MMMT tumors contain epithelial and mesenchymal elements both of which are histologically malignant. The mesenchymal elements may, on the one hand, differentiate towards tissue 'homologous' to the Müllerian tract, such tumors are termed carcinosarcoma, or they may show 'heterologous' tissue foreign to the Müllerian tract. The latter have a lower median survival.

The progression of these tumors tends to be rapid and survival is infrequent even in stage I tumors. The surgical management is as for malignant epithelial tumors followed by adjuvant combination chemotherapy.

Lymphomas

Ovarian involvement by malignant lymphomas is rare except as a manifestation of disseminated nodal lymphoma.

14

Gestational trophoblastic disease

J. Nevin

INTRODUCTION

Gestational trophoblastic disease (GTD) is a spectrum of heterogeneous conditions which arise from products of conception and which may threaten the health and livelihood of young women. Although uncommon, its importance lies in the need for early recognition if treatment is to be translated into cure and continued fertility. It is a health hazard which must be included in the differential diagnosis of a wide variety of clinical conditions.

CLASSIFICATION

Because the spectrum is wide and heterogeneous, there have been several attempts to classify GTD. These were handicapped by the plethora of terms which have been applied to this disease and the diversity of diagnostic tools available.

The World Health Organization (WHO) in 1983 distinguished hydatidiform moles from gestational trophoblastic tumors (Fig. 14.1).

Hydatidiform moles can be complete or partial but the former are more common. Both present as a complication of pregnancy.

Gestational trophoblastic tumors present either consequent to or seemingly unrelated to a pregnancy (molar, abortion or term). The former is likely to be an invasive mole and the latter likely to be a choriocarcinoma. Reliable distinction can only be achieved histologically and this is rarely possible.

COMPLETE HYDATIDIFORM MOLE

This entity is characterized by the absence of a fetus and a uterus filled by grossly swollen avascular villi made up of edematous stroma sur-

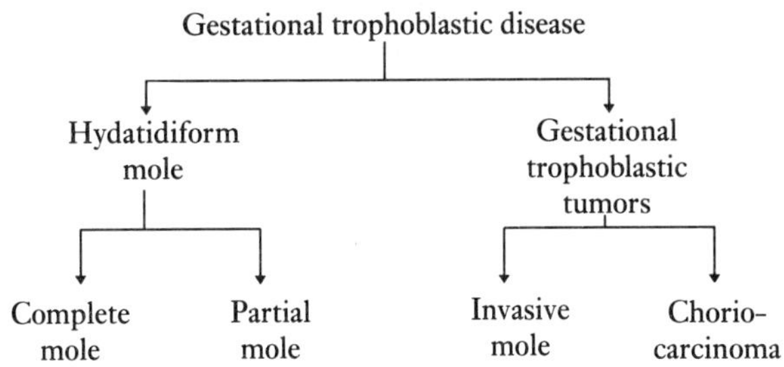

Fig. 14.1 Gestational trophoblastic disease.

rounded by hyperplastic syncytiotrophoblast. The incidence, which is difficult to determine and varies geographically, is approximately 1 per 1000 live births. Genetically usually diploid.

Symptomatology

Patients with hydatidiform mole present as a complication of an existing pregnancy, with a background of amenorrhea, symptoms of pregnancy and a positive pregnancy test. The presenting symptoms can be bleeding, passage of 'grape-like products' or hyperemesis gravidarum (30%). Pain is not a dominant symptom.

Clinical signs

These patients are usually well with no overt distress or hemodynamic compromize but they may be pale. If hyperemesis is present, there may be signs of dehydration and ketosis.

In 65% of patients, uterine examination will reveal a fundal height discordant with gestational age. The consistency of the uterus is 'doughy' rather than cystic.

Vaginal examination may confirm bleeding or a dilated cervix with vesicular products of conception in the vagina.

Twenty per cent of patients will show features of pre-eclampsia. Hypertensive proteinuria before 20 weeks of pregnancy should raise the possibility of a diagnosis of gestational trophoblastic disease. More unusually (10%), hyperthyroidism may manifest as clinical thyrotoxicosis.

Diagnosis and investigation

The ultrasound appearance of an enlarged uterus with echolucent 'black holes surrounded by a rim of white' is absolutely specific.

Abdominal X-ray may provide useful information (an absent fetal skeleton and excessive opacification in the region of the uterine shadow) but if ultrasonography is not available, patients with suspected molar disease, if at all possible, should be referred to an institution with this facility. Pelvic angiography and amniography are specific but excessively invasive.

Extensive investigation for metastatic disease is not appropriate and should be limited to a chest X-ray. A baseline serum beta-HCG and blood count are important.

Treatment

Evacuation of a hydatidiform mole by suction curettage has proved superior to hysterectomy and medical methods. If the uterine size is greater than an equivalent 14 week pregnancy, the evacuation is best guided by ultrasonology. This prevents perforation of the uterine fundus (which is notoriously soft) and ensures that the uterus is adequately emptied.

Brisk bleeding should always be anticipated and transfusion may be necessary. An intravenous infusion of oxytocin should be used to enhance myometrial contractility.

Curettings should always be sent for histology as evidence of choriocarcinoma justifies adjuvant chemotherapy.

Rarely is a hysterectomy necessary for life-threatening hemorrhage or uterine perforation.

Follow-up

Repeat evacuation is not necessary unless bleeding occurs.

Follow-up is dependent on regular monitoring of serum beta-HCG levels. Until levels return to normal, this should be performed every 2 weeks. Thereafter, monthly assays are adequate and should be repeated until the beta-HCG remains below 10 IU for 1 year.

During this interval adequate contraception is essential since an intervening pregnancy will interfere with follow-up and prevent timeous diagnosis of persistent disease.

Any subsequent pregnancy requires an early ultrasound to detect a recurrent hydatidiform mole.

Prognosis

For 80% of patients with a hydatidiform mole, suction curettage is adequate; 20% will develop persistent disease and require further intervention.

The risk of recurrent molar disease after one hydatidiform mole is increased 6–10-fold but is not a contraindication to fertility.

POST-MOLAR GESTATIONAL TROPHOBLASTIC TUMOR (PERSISTENT HYDATIDIFORM MOLE)

The 10–20% of patients with newly diagnosed molar disease will ultimately require therapy additional to curettage. Persistent disease is due either to invasion by molar disease or to the presence *ab initio* of choriocarcinoma with its propensity to invade and metastasize.

Diagnosis and investigation

Persistent hydatidiform mole is usually diagnosed if postevacuation beta-HCG persists (beyond 6–8 weeks), plateaus or increases. Uncommonly compliance with molar follow-up is poor and patients may present at later stages with symptoms and signs related to persistent uterine disease or tumor that has metastasized.

Extensive screening for metastatic disease is probably not cost-effective in the first instance and can be limited to a chest X-ray, biochemistry for liver metastases and ultrasonology of the pelvis. If any of these investigations indicate extrauterine disease, CNS metastases should be excluded by computerized tomography if available and upper abdominal ultrasonology used to assess kidneys and spleen. These last-mentioned investigations are also necessary if beta-HCG levels are high (>40 000 IU) or the interval between preceding pregnancy and chemotherapy exceeds 4 months.

Lumbar puncture for CSF assay of beta-HCG levels is only performed where indicated.

Treatment of persistent hydatidiform mole

Repeat evacuation is advisable if ultrasonology suggests retained products of conception. This procedure carries the risk of Asherman's syndrome and should be undertaken cautiously.

Chemotherapy forms the mainstay of treatment and response is measured by beta-HCG assay (Chapter 15).

Contraception is important.

In patients with completed families and no evidence of metastatic disease or in whom a chemoresistant nidus appears to be uterine, there is a role for hysterectomy. If levels persist after this surgery, chemotherapy is necessary.

Prognosis

Of those patients with persistent hydatidiform mole, 99% will be cured by chemotherapy and/or surgery.

Management

Management is summarized in Fig. 14.2.

PARTIAL HYDATIDIFORM MOLE

This entity is characterized by the presence of a fetus, albeit abnormal, and a placenta consisting of focal areas of hydatid change interspersed within normal tissue. Abortion usually occurs although the occasional partial mole reaches term and a triploid infant is delivered.

Gestational trophoblastic tumor rarely follows a partial molar pregnancy but should be excluded by beta-HCG follow-up. There is not the same need for prolonged contraception as in complete molar disease; once levels have normalized fertility can be pursued.

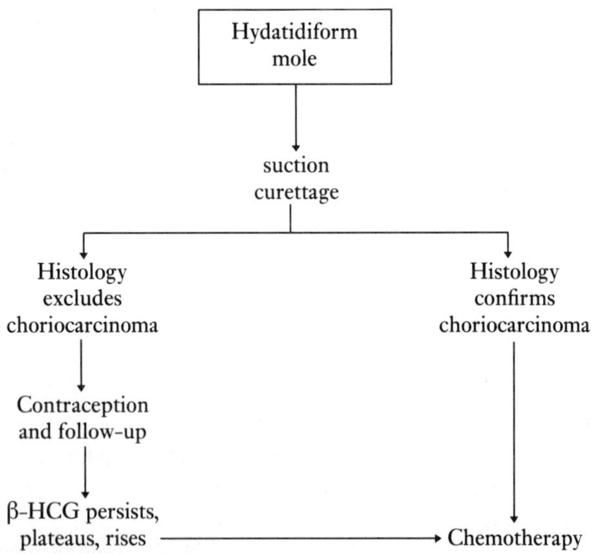

Fig. 14.2 Management of hydatidiform mole.

GESTATIONAL TROPHOBLASTIC TUMOR: CHORIOCARCINOMA

The difference between hydatidiform mole and choriocarcinoma lies in their relationship to pregnancy. It has been emphasized that hydatidiform mole complicates an existing pregnancy. Choriocarcinoma manifests after a preceding pregnancy.

Clinical features

The preceding pregnancy might have been a hydatidiform mole (60%), an abortion (20%), a normal full-term pregnancy (15%) or an ectopic pregnancy (5%). In the developing world it is sometimes difficult to elicit a history of the index pregnancy.

The uterus may contain residual tumor and give rise to vaginal bleeding and a pelvic mass.

However, patients may have symptoms and signs related to their metastatic disease. In order of decreasing frequency, the viscera (with related symptoms and signs) most commonly affected are lung (hemoptysis), vagina (bleeding and nodules, particularly in the suburethral region), brain (convulsions, altered levels of consciousness and localizing signs), liver (right hypocondrial pain and tenderness), kidney (hematuria), bowel (rectal bleeding and melena) and spleen (pain).

Generalized symptoms related to widespread metastatic disease (weight loss, fatigue and poor appetite) may be present. If the beta-HCG levels are high enough to exert a significant thyrotropic effect, thyrotoxicosis will manifest.

From the above description it is obvious that many of the features of choriocarcinoma are non-gynecological and this explains why 80% of these patients present initially to other disciplines. This may contribute to the delay in diagnosis, since non-gynecological practitioners may fail to draw the appropriate association.

Diagnosis

Assays for beta-HCG play a pivotal role.

It is usual and even preferable for histology to play no part in the diagnosis of choriocarcinoma. Vaginal biopsy characteristically results in catastrophic bleeding and should be avoided. Ultrasonology has very little role except in excluding an intrauterine pregnancy.

In the developing world, detecting beta-HCG can be achieved by using standard urinary pregnancy tests. By repeating the test in dilution it is possible, with minimal facilities, to estimate the levels of urinary beta-HCG.

Special investigations

A search for metastatic disease is mandatory. Every patient should have a chest X-ray, computerized tomography of the brain and ultrasonography of the liver, kidneys, spleen and pelvis.

Pelvic angiography has a small role in searching for adnexal metastases and is useful in confirming that the disease is confined to the uterus.

Thyroid function tests will identify patients in whom thyroid suppression is required as an interim measure until the thyrotropic stimulus has abated.

Prognosis

There is no malignancy with a better outcome. More than 90% of these patients can expect to be cured and most of them will be left with fertility intact.

Therapy

Chemotherapy has revolutionized the treatment of these patients and for countless women has reversed the once inevitable path to death.

Most tumors are chemosensitive but as experience with malignant GTD has evolved, it has become obvious that response to chemotherapy is not uniform and that variable regimens are required. Patients with less aggressive disease need simpler treatment. Those in whom the disease is likely to prove chemoresistant require more drastic intervention *ab initio*. Regimens are discussed in Chapter 15 on chemotherapy.

Progress is monitored by serial measurements of serum beta-HCG.

Until levels have been normal for 1 year patients must remain on effective contraception.

Surgery has a limited, albeit important role in the treatment of choriocarcinoma and is largely confined to those patients in whom resistance to chemotherapy occurs. Hysterectomy is useful if the chemoresistant nidus appears to be uterine. Occasionally it may be necessary to resect deposits of chemoresistant tumor in non-gynecological viscera such as brain or lung. Such surgery should only be undertaken where all other options have been attempted.

Where genital bleeding is life threatening or where chemotherapy and surgery have failed to eliminate pelvic tumor deposits, radiotherapy may be useful. Radiotherapy is also used for cerebral metastases and in this context has superseded intrathecal methotrexate. Details are provided in Chapter 16 on radiotherapy.

CONTRACEPTION IN GESTATIONAL TROPHOBLASTIC DISEASE

Monitoring the response of GTD to treatment is dependent on the absence of any other source of beta-HCG. It is therefore mandatory to avoid another pregnancy until beta-HCG levels have been normal for 1 year. Effective contraception forms an integral part of management.

Combined oral contraceptives were thought to prolong beta-HCG response curves and to increase the likelihood of chemotherapeutic intervention. These fears have proved groundless and hormonal contraception, oral or injectable, is the reversible contraception of choice in patients with GTD.

Where there is a possibility of intrauterine neoplasia, it is advisable to avoid an IUCD.

Barrier methods under these circumstances are not sufficiently effective.

15

Chemotherapy for gynecological cancer

C. Falkson and G. Falkson

INTRODUCTION

The basic principles of chemotherapy apply to gynecological malignancies. Before cytostatic drugs are administered histologic classification of the tumor is essential. The therapeutic index (benefit ratio of expected treatment effect relative to expected toxicity) of the drugs in relation to the stage of disease must be determined. The role of cytostatic drug (or hormone) treatment compared with other treatment modalities must be evaluated. Individual patient discriminants such as age, performance status, functional organ reserve and concomitant disease play an important part in both the interdisciplinary management of the patient and in the decisions whether (or which) cytostatic drugs should given.

It is important to emphasize that the rising costs of treatment with cytostatic agents is a cause for concern worldwide. It has become clear that starting with the most effective cytostatic treatment saves money. When these expensive drugs cure or control disease then hospitalization, antibiotics and transfusion costs are reduced. The indirect effects of loss of work and function caused by inadequate treatments are of great economic importance. In developing countries with limited health budgets these problems are amplified and there is a need for cost-effective centralized treatment facilities so that diseases such as choriocarcinoma and ovarian cancer can receive adequate treatment and save resources.

An important function of the medical oncologist is to decide not only when cytostatic drugs should be given but also when they should not be used and when they should be stopped. These decisions, when correctly made, are in the best interest of the patient and of the state. Before any cytostatic treatment is started the infrastructure for such treatment should be in place. This includes properly trained personnel skilled in the administration of cytostatic drugs and facilities for sterile mixing of chemotherapeutic agents.

SQUAMOUS CELL CARCINOMA OF THE CERVIX

Chemotherapy has been reserved for patients whose disease was too advanced to be treated by surgery and/or radiotherapy. Poor kidney function, fistulae and pelvic sepsis in these patients severely restricts cytostatic administration and the therapeutic benefit is limited. Furthermore, cytostatic treatment is poorly tolerated in patients who have previously received therapeutic doses of radiotherapy. Recently an increasing body of evidence has accumulated showing that squamous cell carcinoma of the cervix is sensitive to cytostatic agents.

The response rate to both single agent and combination chemotherapy in squamous cell carcinoma of the cervix is depicted in Table 15.1. None of the single agents with the exception of cisplatinum has shown an acceptable efficacy. The response rate to cisplatinum varies between 23 and 40% with a duration of response of between 4 and 7 months. Different dosage schedules do not seem to alter the results.

The most promising combination chemotherapy regimen appears to be bleomycin, ifosfamide and cisplatinum (BIP) with a reported response rate of 69%. Toxic effects are similar to other combinations. Three courses of BIP are given at intervals of 3 weeks and should be given prior to radiotherapy in advanced carcinoma.

VAGINAL CARCINOMA

Cytostatics have very little effect on primary or recurrent vaginal carcinoma and cisplatinum in contrast to squamous carcinoma of the cervix has no significant activity.

Table 15.1 Chemotherapy for squamous carcinoma of the cervix

Chemotherapy	*Response (%)*
A. Single Agents	
Alkylating Agents, 5-Fluorouracil, Methotrexate Bleomycin, Doxorubicin, Carboplatinum	<20
Ifosfamide	40
Cisplatinum	20–40
B. Combination Chemotherapy	
Bleomycin + Ifosfamide + Cisplatinum	>60
Methotrexate + Vinblastine + Doxorubicin + Cisplatinum	60

VULVAL CARCINOMA

Chemotherapy is mainly used in advanced, irresectable vulval carcinoma with considerable success. Mitomycin C and 5-Fluorouracil are used with concomitant external beam radiotherapy in these patients.

ADENOCARCINOMA OF THE ENDOMETRIUM

Adenocarcinoma of the endometrium treated surgically, with or without postoperative radiotherapy, results in cure rate of 70–80%. Only a small proportion of patients such as those with disseminated disease require further treatment and chemotherapy may play a role in this respect.

The response rates, which have been uniformly disappointing, to both single agent as well as combination chemotherapy can be found in Table 15.2.

Medroxyprogesterone acetate (MPA) (200 and 400 mg daily) has been used extensively with a consistent response rate of up to 40% but its use as an adjuvant agent has not been shown to be of value.

Table 15.2 Chemotherapy for adenocarcinoma of the endometrium

Chemotherapy	*Response (%)*	*Median survival (months)*
A. Single Agent		
Vinblastine, Cyclophosphamide 5-Fluorouracil		<20
Carboplatinum, Doxorubicin, 4-Epidoxorubicin, Hexamethylmelamine		<30
Medroxyprogesterone Acetate only in Advanced Disease		20–40
Cisplatinum		4–46
B. Combination Chemotherapy		
Medroxyprogesterone Acetate only in Advanced Disease + Cyclophosphamide + Doxorubicin + 5-Fluorouracil	22	<7
Methotrexate + Vinblastine + Doxorubicin + Cyclophosphamide	60	9
Cyclophosphamide + Doxorubicin + Cisplatinum	30–60	<18

EPITHELIAL OVARIAN CARCINOMA

First-line treatment

Chemotherapy plays an important role in the treatment of all patients with epithelial ovarian carcinoma except in stages Ia and Ib with well or moderately differentiated histology. In patients with adequately staged Ic and II disease good results (up to 77% for 5 year survival) are seen with adjuvant cisplatinum-based combination chemotherapy. It is important to stress that in patients with ovarian cancer exposure to any cytostatic treatment significantly decreases the chance of response to subsequent treatment so that the decision about initial cytostatic treatment is critical.

In advanced ovarian carcinoma a number of high risk factors have been identified. These include, residual disease after primary surgery, age, performance status and grade of the primary tumor.

Depending on these risk factors, the 3 year survival rate in stage IIIa–IV is between 7 and 60%. The efficacy of single agent chemotherapy in advanced disease is depicted in Table 15.3. The response rate to these agents varies between 35 and 65% with a medium survival time of approximately 1 year. Five to 10% of women with advanced ovarian cancer can be cured with single alkylating agents such as Melphalan. There is still a place for single alkylating agents in frail elderly patients, but this is not recommended for patients with adequate organ reserve who can tolerate the therapeutic dose of a platinum compound.

Table 15.3 Chemotherapy for advanced epithelial ovarian cancer: commonly used agents and combinations

Agent(s)	*Response (%)*	*Median survival (months)*
Melphalan	11–54	14–28
Cyclophosphamide	21–67	11–12
Cisplatinum	13–71	20–23
Carboplatinum	53–57	–
Cisplatinum + Cyclophosphamide	59–76	18–36
Carboplatinum + Cyclophosphamide	73	18
Cisplatinum + Adriamycin + Cyclophosphamide	51–81	16–36
Hexamethylmelamine + Cyclophosphamide + Adriamycin + 5-Fluorouracil	76	29

Platinum compounds have shown high activity in cancer of the ovary and the 10 year survival rates have doubled with cisplatinum-based chemotherapy.

Combination chemotherapy was shown to be better than single-agent chemotherapy using the four drug combination hexamethylmelamine, cyclophosphamide, adriamycin and 5-fluorouracil (Hexa-CAF). The response rate was better than melphalan (75% vs 54%) with twice as many complete remissions and longer medium survival (29 vs 17 months); however the toxicity with Hexa-CAF is significant.

Cisplatinum has emerged as the most active drug in multiagent chemotherapy and it seems that high doses may be most effective if given in first line.

Since the early 1980s two cisplatinum-based combinations have been used with good response rates and acceptable toxicity. These are PAC (cisplatinum, adriamycin and cyclophosphamide) with response rates varying between 51 and 81% and a median survival of 16–36 months and PC (cisplatinum and cyclophosphamide) with response rates varying between 50 and 76% and median survival rates between 18 and 36 months (Table 15.3).

Because of the potential cardiotoxicity of adriamycin, PC has become the reference arm of several ongoing randomized trials.

Carboplatin has emerged in the last decade as an active drug in combination treatment for patients with advanced ovarian cancer. Although the efficacy of carboplatin has not been shown to be superior to cisplatinum it has substantially less tendency to cause nausea and vomiting, neurotoxicity and nephrotoxicity.

Taxol, which is derived from the bark of the western Yew, has definite activity in ovarian cancer and the results of studies presently in progress will be watched with interest.

Second-line treatment

The results of second-line treatment with current chemotherapy regimens have been disappointing. Carboplatin has activity in patients previously treated with cisplatinum but the response is subject to the relative resistance to cisplatinum. The most promising new development has been the activity shown by taxol in recurrent ovarian cancers, which has been shown to be active in cisplatinum-resistant disease.

The efficacy of intraperitoneal chemotherapy, despite more than three decades experience and the publication of many uncontrolled studies, has not been proven to be efficacious in the primary treatment of patients with epithelial ovarian carcinoma.

NON-EPITHELIAL OVARIAN CARCINOMA

1. Germ cell tumors
   (a) Non-dysgerminoma. Combination chemotherapy is recommended for all patients irrespective of stage with non-dysgerminomatous germ cell tumors. A number of combinations have been used including vicristine, actinomycin D and cyclophosphamide (VAC), cisplatinum, vincristine and bleomycin (PVB) and cisplatinum, etoposide and bleomycin (PEB). The latter combination has shown excellent activity and acceptable toxicity with 98% of patients having complete remission.

   A positive serum tumor marker (alpha-fetoprotein, beta-HCG) should be used as a guideline for cytostatic treatment. Where no tumor marker is present a second-look laparotomy should be considered to assess the efficacy of cytostatic treatment.

   (b) Pure dysgerminoma. The cure rate of stage I pure dysgerminoma is high with a 91% 5 year survival rate. In more advanced disease the response rate to chemotherapy is 83–90%, using the same combinations as for non-dysgerminomatous germ cell tumors.
2. Stromal cell tumors. Advanced granulosa cell tumors may respond to combination chemotherapy including cisplatinum, bleomycin and vinblastine. Medroxyprogesterone acetate may also have therapeutic activity.

GESTATIONAL TROPHOBLASTIC DISEASE

One of the success stories of cytostatic treatment is the cure rate achieved in gestational trophoblastic disease (GTD) which usually affects young women.

Both the life-threatening nature of GTD and the potential curability make it imperative that all patients are referred to centers where sufficient expertise exists for correct treatment.

All types of trophoblastic disease produce human chorionic gonadotrophin (HCG) and its beta-chain in proportion to the volume of disease. Disease response should under all circumstances, with or without chemotherapy, be monitored using this extremely useful tumor marker.

GTD has been discussed in Chapter 14. The majority (80%) of patients with hydatidiform mole need no further treatment provided that weekly beta-HCG assays can be performed until the titer returns to normal. Criteria which indicate the need for chemotherapy in GTD include beta-HCG serum levels exceeding 20 000 units/ml persisting 4 weeks after evacuation, increasing beta-HCG serum levels and the histologic identification of choriocarcinoma. All patients with distant metastases should be treated with chemotherapy.

Patients requiring cytostatic treatment for trophoblastic disease can be divided into low, medium and high risk groups. In order to classify these patients the WHO scoring system is used (Table 15.4).

Patients will fall into one of three categories (Table 15.4): low (0–4), medium (5–7) or high risk (>8). Recent opinion suggests that patients with scores greater than 12 should be viewed as ultra high risk and accorded special attention.

1. Low risk patients (0–4). Single agent treatment is adequate to cure more than 90% of patients with low risk GTD. Methotrexate combined with folinic acid or actinomycin D are usually used.

   The slope of beta-HCG decrease should be carefully recorded to monitor the efficacy of chemotherapy. When the beta-HCG serum level is below 10 units/ml one or two insurance courses are given.
2. Medium risk patients (5–7). All medium risk patients should receive combination chemotherapy. A number of combinations have been used with success. A commonly used combination includes etoposide, methotrexate, actinomycin D, cyclophosphamide and vincristine (EMA-CO).

   Serum beta-HCG should be monitored as in low risk patients.
3. High risk patients (>8). For high risk patients EMA-CO should also be used but failing this a combination containing cisplatinum, etoposide, bleomycin and ifosfamide have been used successfully.

Table 15.4 WHO scoring system for gestational trophoblastic disease

Score	*0*	*1*	*2*	*4*
Age (years)	≤39	>39		
Antecedent pregnancy	mole	abortion	term	
Beta-HCG (IU/litre)	$<10^3$	10^3–10^4	10^4–10^5	$>10^5$
Interval (months)	<4	4–6	7–12	>12
Largest tumor (cm)		3–5	>5	
Site of metastases		spleen/kidney	GIT/liver	brain
Number of metastases		1–4	4–8	>8
Prior chemotherapy			single drug	2 or more drugs

4. Ultra high risk patients (>8). There is a predictable and significant percentage of patients in this group who will fail to respond to conventional multiagent chemotherapy. Of these, some will respond to platinum combination chemotherapy. It has been suggested, but never proven, that these patients should have first-line platinum combination chemotherapy as in the high risk group. At this stage it is probably prudent to follow the same treatment strategy as for patients in the high risk group, i.e. induce treatment with EMA-CO and resort to the above mentioned platinum combination in case of failure.

CHEMOTHERAPY AND SIDE-EFFECTS

A wide range of side-effects may occur in patients receiving treatment (Table 15.5). Side-effects are often related to dose and duration of treatment and may also be enhanced in combination treatment. Thorough knowledge of drug interactions is imperative before embarking on chemotherapy.

Table 15.5 Chemotherapeutic agents: incidence of side-effects

	Bone marrow	Phlebitis sclerosant	Neurological	Skin	Pulmonary	Renal	Hepatic	Cardiac	Endocrine	Bladder	Gut	Allergic	Alopecia	Metabolic	Nausea/Vomiting	Stomatitis
A. Methotrexate	***		*	*	*	*	**				***		*		*	***
5-Fluorouracil	***		*	*							**		*		*	***
Cyclophosphamide	***			*			*	*	*	**	**		**	*	**	
B. Leukeran	***		*	*	*		*								*	
Melphalan	***										*				**	
Actinomycin D	***	*	*	*							**		**	*	**	*
Adriamycin	***	**	*					**			**		**		**	**
C. Bleomycin	*		**	***	***		*					*			**	*
Mitomycin C	***	*									*				**	
D. Vinblastine	*	*											*			
Vincristine	*	*	***				*						*	*		
Etoposide	***	*														
E. Cisplatinum	*		*			***									**	
Carboplatinum	***		*			*									*	*

A. = Nucleic acid and folate antimetabolites; B. = Alkylating agents; C. = Antibiotics; D. = Vinca alkaloids; E. = miscellaneous.

Nausea and vomiting are common and among the most distressing side-effects of chemotherapy. A wide range of anti-emetics is available to treat these side-effects. They include among others metoclopramide, dexamethasone and lorazepam. Recently the introduction of 5-HT antagonists has proven to be an extremely effective albeit costly medication against nausea and vomiting.

16

Radiotherapy for gynecological cancer

L. van Wijk

INTRODUCTION

Radiotherapy plays a significant role in both curative treatment and palliation of gynecology cancer. The radiotherapist should have a close working relationship with gynecological colleagues to ensure that patients are referred with the necessary information to enable correct staging and treatment decisions. Except for gestational trophoblastic disease, a histologic diagnosis in imperative.

In this chapter a few tennets of radiotherapy are introduced as well as its application in gynecological cancers. Lastly, some of the problems that beset radiotherapy in developing countries are examined.

BASIC ASPECTS OF RADIOTHERAPY

1. Units of radiotherapy. The amount of radiation energy absorbed in a medium, e.g. tissues is described by the Gray (Gy), defined as that dose of radiation producing absorption of 1 joule of energy per kg of tissue. Previously the unit was the rad (= 0.1 J/kg, i.e. 100 rads = 1 Gy).
2. The biological effects of absorption of photon energy in tissue leads to ejection of orbital electrons from atoms or molecules (= ionization). The ejected or secondary electrons produce further ionized atoms. The critical intracellular target of ionizing radiation damage is probably the DNA molecule.

   Tumors can outgrow their blood supply resulting in necrotic areas. A zone of relatively hypoxic cells exists between the anoxic zones and well-oxygenated cells closer to blood vessels. A dose of photon radiation has to be increased threefold to kill the same number of hypoxic than oxygenated cells. In everyday clinical practice the only intervention possible to minimize tumor cell hypoxia is to reverse severe anemia prior to radiotherapy treatment.

Conventional radiotherapy empirically developed fractionated schemes or daily increments of radiation given five times per week at 1.8–2 Gy per fraction over a period of several weeks. Radiocurability of such protracted treatment is far superior to a single treatment and a much higher total dose can be administered by a fractionated scheme.

3. Teletherapy. Also known as external beam radiotherapy (EBRT). Photon radiation is used most commonly.

   The following megavoltage units are in common use:

   (a) Cobalt 60 – units emit gamma rays of average energy 1.25 mV. Cobalt units are durable, practical and relatively cheap compared with modern X-ray units.
   (b) Megavoltage X-ray units or linear accelerators (linacs). Electrons are accelerated towards a target through voltage differences of 4–30 million volts, depending on the energy of X-rays required. The greater penetration of the higher energies is most suited to treating deep-seated tumors, especially in obese patients.

4. Brachytherapy. A radioactive isotope is placed in close proximity to a tumor either by implanting the source within or around the tumor (interstitial brachytherapy) or within a cavity such as the uterus or vagina (intracavitary therapy = ICT). There is a rapid fall-off in intensity of radiation away from the sources with relative sparing of surrounding tissues or organs, hence the designation brachytherapy (therapy over short distance). In gynecological ICT, the sources are loaded into special containers or applicators. In older methods, sources are manually preloaded into the applicators which are then inserted into an anesthetized patient. This method has many drawbacks. In after-loaded systems, the applicators are inserted empty and satisfactory position confirmed. The sources are then after-loaded either manually or remotely controlled.

   Two broad groups of isotopes are employed in gynecological ICT depending on the source activity or dose rate. Low dose rate (LDR), either radium or caesium. High dose rate (HDR) isotopes, either iridium or cobalt, cannot be handled manually and are inserted via remote after-loading systems (RALS).

   Many gynecological applicators for cervical cancer have been developed; most consist of an intrauterine tube or tandem and two oval-shaped containers placed in each lateral vaginal fornix (vaginal colpostats or ovoids). In the Manchester technique three tandem lengths and three ovoid sizes were developed. Owing to the large differential of dose across the pelvis, two dosage reference points were chosen. Manchester point A lies 2 cm lateral from the center of the tandem and 2 cm superior to the lateral fornix. Point B lies 3 cm lateral to point A. Radium or caesium loading varies with tandem length or ovoid size in a predetermined manner so that the dose rate at point A remains relatively constant at 0.5 ± 10% Gy/hour.

In HDR-RALS, sources enter the applicators as a pre-arranged source 'train', or a single source is moved in a stepwise fashion to deliver the desired dose distribution.

Although the basic principles of gynecological brachytherapy were developed with preloaded radium sources, the trend has been to replace radium in LDR work with cesium-137.

5. Inverse square law. If radiation dose is measured over a fixed area closer and further away from a source, the intensity at any given point is inversely proportional to the square of the distance between the said area and the source (i.e. dose = $1/D^2$). The inverse square law has important clinical applications.
6. Skin sparing. In modern megavoltage teletherapy, maximum energy absorption is below the skin surface, and severe reactions are rare. In the treatment of pelvic tumors, the skin of the gluteal folds and perineal area is perpendicular to the beam, while skin may also be buried under folds in obese patients. In these areas, skin sparing is not possible and significant irritation may occur and be aggravated by moisture and friction.
7. Treatment planning. A decision to treat with radiotherapy sets in motion the treatment planning process. Ideally a maximally tolerated radiation dose is delivered to the tumor and a surrounding volume of tissue at risk of neoplastic infiltration or lymphatic spread (the 'target volume'), while minimizing exposure to dose-limiting normal organs. In pelvic malignancies these are the rectosigmoid, bladder, distal ureters, as well as small bowel loops within the true pelvis. Vaginal dose also needs to be considered where ICT is used. It is impossible to avoid castration as the ovaries are highly radiosensitive.

   Decisions need to be made concerning:
8. Intent of radiotherapy in cancer treatment
   (a) Curative or 'radical' radiotherapy. A protracted course of fractionated treatment is given with the aim of curing the disease in a patient without known distant metastases.
   (b) Palliative. The aim is the alleviation of symptoms and not primarily to prolong life. Where disease is incurable due to the presence of distant metastases, advanced local disease or poor physical condition of the patient, relief of pain, vaginal discharge or bleeding etc. is possible with a short course of radio-

therapy. Patients with incurable cancer who are asymptomatic do not need palliative irradiation. One or a few large fractions are given. Acute reactions are minimized and the potential for late morbidity produced by large fractions is not realized due to the short survival of these patients.

(c) Adjuvant radiotherapy is used postoperatively in the radical treatment of patients, aiming to sterilize microscopic deposits (either known or surmised) in a tumor bed or regional lymphatics. The aim is improvement of locoregional tumor control.

The role of radiotherapy in specific gynecological cancers is as follows.

CERVICAL CANCER

Curative radiotherapy

The dose of fractionated radiotherapy to sterilize 90% of microscopic deposits from epithelial tumors is 50 Gy, i.e. also the minimum dose to be administered to the pelvic lymph nodes at risk in cervical carcinoma. Larger, clinically apparent tumors require 60–80 Gy which is beyond the tolerance of normal pelvic organs. The uterus, however, is relatively radioresistant, allowing intracavitary therapy to deliver, usually in conjunction with EBRT, doses of up to 85 Gy to the paracervical tissues. Due to the rapid fall-off of dose, ICT alone cannot deliver tumoricidal doses to the lateral parametrium or iliac nodes. The main contribution of the 50–60 Gy needed in these areas comes from EBRT.

In early stage disease the emphasis is on ICT supplying tumoricidal doses to the known centrally situated tumor. As only about 20% of the dose at point A will be received by lateral tissue from ICT, EBRT is used to supplement the dose to the sidewall regions.

In more advanced tumor, with parametrial involvement and high risk of nodal spread, the emphasis is on EBRT to the whole pelvis to a dose of 50–55 Gy, followed by ICT supplementing the dose to the central tumor. This sequence allows tumor shrinkage, enabling closer application of sources and improved doses to the periphery of the tumor. Extensive residual parametrial involvement at the end of treatment can be 'boosted' by EBRT of reduced portal size. Routinely extending the superior portal limit above L5–S1 interface to include upper common iliac or para-aortic nodes increases morbidity and is not recommended. In the treatment suggestions given below, ICT doses are for radium sources.

1. Stage IB + IIA. While results for radical surgery and radiotherapy are identical, surgical expertise may be unavailable or the patient physically unsuitable for surgery. Surgery may be untenable in extremely bulky tumors or stage IIA with extensive vaginal involvement. Whole pelvis EBRT is given at 2 Gy per fraction, 5 times per week with parallel opposed portals (POP) or preferably with a four-field box arrangement; 40–45 Gy is given over 4–5 weeks, followed by two or three ICT insertions. Pelvic sidewall doses should reach a total of 50–55 Gy. The dose to point A should be 75–80 Gy. Alternatively, in small tumors ICT is given first, weekly for three insertions. Sidewall doses are then supplemented with POP and shielding of central structures.

   In frail elderly patients, unlikely to tolerate a full course of treatment as described, and where the tumor is of small diameter, three insertions without EBRT should suffice.
2. Stage IIB + IIIB. Whole pelvis EBRT to 54 Gy is followed by a single LDR insertion. Total point A doses of 75 Gy should be reached.

   The dose to the anterior rectal wall from ICT can be measured at insertion by means of a rectal probe or estimated from lateral X-rays corrected for magnification. A rule of thumb is to limit total (EBRT + ICT) anterior rectal wall doses to 65 Gy or less in older patients. High measured rectal doses may necessitate shorter than planned insertion times of ICT sources.
3. Stage IV. Stage IVA – fit patients with relatively low volume tumor should be treated 'radically' as in stage IIIB as occasional cures are possible. The majority of patients, however, will have advanced local tumor and poor performance status. Cure probability is remote and palliative radiation is given. Surgical diversion of fecal or urinary stream is offered, if the service is available, in patients with fistulae (Chapter 5).

   Stage IVB. See palliative irradiation below.

Adjuvant postoperative radiotherapy

Recommended after:

1. Radical hysterectomy with poor prognostic factors: tumor diameter >4 cm with deep stromal invasion (especially if endothelial-lined space invasion is present), parametrial extension, resection lines involved or <3 mm from tumor, or metastatic pelvic nodes.
2. Simple hysterectomy for benign conditions with 'occult' carcinoma found histologically.

Dose per fraction is 1.8 Gy, five times per week to 50.4 Gy. Except for the indication of positive pelvic lymph nodes, the vaginal vault should be boosted with ICT, either a pair of ovoids or an apically loaded vaginal cylinder. Adjuvant pelvic radiation has not unequivocally been shown to improve survival although it significantly reduces pelvic failures.

Palliative irradiation

Patients with stage IV (or advanced pelvic tumor, poor performance status or renal failure) are offered palliative treatment if symptoms are present. A common regimen is 3 Gy for 10 fractions via shortened POP. Symptomatic metastatic sites, e.g. para-aortic lymphadenopathy, are best treated with POP, 3 Gy for eight to ten fractions. Painful bony metastases may respond to a single fraction of 8–10 Gy.

Special management problems

1. Carcinoma of the cervix in pregnancy
   (a) With viable fetus (more than 24 weeks). Patients are delivered by cesarian section as soon as fetal viability is reached. In stage IB and early stage IIA a radical hysterectomy and pelvic lymphadenectomy is performed at the time of cesarian section. If radical surgery is impossible or advanced stage tumor present, radiotherapy commences 10 days after cesarian section in the usual manner.
   (b) With non-viable fetus (less than 24 weeks) stage IB and IIA. Radical hysterectomy and pelvic lymphadenectomy is the preferred treatment. If surgery is not possible or more advanced disease is present, radiotherapy is started with whole pelvis EBRT. In the first trimester, spontaneous abortion is allowed to occur. In the second trimester, a hysterotomy is performed after 20–30 Gy to prevent the aborting of a large fetus through a diseased cervix. After hysterotomy, RT proceeds in the usual manner.
2. Recurrent carcinoma of cervix. Pelvic recurrences after radical hysterectomy should be treated radically with 1.8 Gy fives times per week to 50.4 Gy, followed by vaginal cylinder ICT if central recurrence or small volume boosts if lateral recurrence. Recurrences after previous radiation are rarely amenable to any salvage procedures and are treated symptomatically.
3. Carcinoma of the cervix in the elderly. In fit patients over 70 years

of age, the tendency to give a short palliative course of radiotherapy should be resisted and those with good performance status and without other life-shortening disease should be offered radical radiotherapy.

UTERINE CORPUS CANCER

Endometrial carcinoma

CURATIVE RADIOTHERAPY

Surgery is the corner stone of treatment and should always be undertaken unless contraindicated by serious medical contraindications. Two methods of primary radiotherapy are available:

1. In stage I–II, Heyman's procedure involves the tight packing of metal pellets (each loaded with 10 mg of radium) into the uterine cavity under general or spinal anesthesia. Two insertions are performed 3 weeks apart, each delivering approximately 30 Gy at 1 cm from the endometrial surface.
2. Stage I–III. In less obese patients, whole pelvis EBRT, 2 Gy for 25 fractions, followed by two insertions with tandem and ovoids 1 week apart, to deliver a summated dose of 80 Gy to point A.

ADJUVANT POSTOPERATIVE IRRADIATION (STAGE I–II)

The standard treatment of endometrial carcinoma is TAH and BSO. There are as many proponents of preoperative as of postoperative radiotherapy. The trend is towards the latter as patients can be better selected for adjuvant pelvic radiotherapy on the basis of surgical findings and adverse histologic prognostic factors 30% risk of pelvic nodal metastases (Chapter 12).

INDICATIONS ARE

1. Grade 3 lesions.
2. More than half myometrial invasion, any grade.
3. Adenosquamous or clear cell histology.
4. Grade 2, less than 50% invasion but over 2 cm tumor diameter.
5. Stage II. These patients receive whole pelvis irradiation (4–6 weeks

postoperatively) preferably with a four-field technique, 1.8 Gy five times per week to 50.4 Gy, followed by insertion of a vaginal cylinder delivering a further 20 Gy to the vaginal mucosa.

Patients with grade 1 tumors involving more than one-third but less than one-half of the myometrium, on grade 2 less than 50% penetration and under 2 cm in diameter are at low risk for pelvic lymph node spread although they have a 10–15% risk of vaginal relapse. A vaginal cylinder insertion 6–8 weeks postoperatively (delivering 60 Gy to the vaginal epithelium) reduces this likehood to less than 5%. Patients with grade 1 tumor with less than one-third invasion do not require adjuvant treatment.

Patients with recurrence in the pelvis after previous TAH and BSO should receive whole pelvis EBRT and a vaginal cylinder as for adjuvant postoperative radiotherapy. About half of these patients are salvageable with RT.

6. Stage III and IVA. Where the diagnosis of stage III is made postoperatively (e.g. ovarian micrometastases), the prognosis is reasonable if postoperative radiotherapy is added. Where other pelvic structures are involved, the prognosis is generally poor even with radical pelvic irradiation. The selection of patients for radical or palliative RT is individualized.

Leiomyosarcoma of the uterus

Since residual pelvic masses after surgery and local recurrences are notoriously radioresistant, routine adjuvant pelvic radiotherapy after TAH is not recommended. The high risk of distant metastatic relapse also negates adjuvant RT. Symptomatic patients are considered for palliative RT or a trial of chemotherapy.

Malignant mixed Müllerian sarcomas

Although the role of adjuvant radiotherapy is controversial, these tumors are more radiosensitive than the leiomyosarcomas and hence there is a case for adjuvant pelvic radiotherapy. The high risk of distal relapse can be reduced by, for example four cycles of cisplatinum – Adriamycin chemotherapy postoperatively, followed by radiotherapy as described for endometrial carcinoma.

CARCINOMA OF THE VAGINA

Whole pelvis EBRT (50–55 Gy) and vaginal cylinder ICT is indicated delivering 20 Gy to the vagina mucosa.

CARCINOMA OF THE OVARY

Radiotherapy is infrequently used except for palliative irradiation of recurrent, symptomatic pelvic masses or metastatic sites. Adjuvant radiotherapy for stage IC and stage IA or B grade 3 (or even in stage II–III where debulking to a microscopic residium has been achieved) is acceptable if chemotherapy cannot be administered. The technique is simple and does not require elaborate planning procedures although a simulator or image intensifier is required to localize the entire abdominal cavity. EBRT is given through POP to the whole abdomen, followed by pelvic boost.

CARCINOMA OF THE VULVA

Postoperative radiotherapy

The vulva should be irradiated if resection lines are less than 8 mm from the tumor edge. The groin and ipsilateral hemipelvis are irradiated if more than two groin nodes are positive, extracapsular nodal spread is found or if a macroscopic metastases (more than 5 mm) is present in a single node. A dose of 50.4 Gy is given at 1.8 Gy per fraction through POP to the nodal and/or vulval sites. Where the primary site is irradiated, skin reactions in the perineal area may necessitate 1–2 weeks of treatment interruption although healing is usually complete afterwards.

Advanced vulval carcinoma

Ultraradical surgery may be untenable in advanced disease if sphincter function is compromized by surgery. Alternatively, groin nodes may be fixed or ulcerated. Disease control can be achieved by the simple excision of bulky mobile groin nodes, followed by irradiation through POP in conjunction with a 4 day constant infusion of 5-fluorouracil, 1 g/m^2/day during the first and fourth week of radiotherapy. Mitomycin C 10 mg/kg intravenously is given on day 1 only; 2 Gy per fraction is administered to the pelvis, five times per week from L5–S1 to at least 2 cm below the vulval tumor. The portals are made wide enough to encompass the groin nodes. Appropriate shielding is used to screen out normal tissues. A brisk perineal radiation reaction (wet desquamation) may necessitate a 1–2 week rest period. If good regression is noted, EBRT is stopped at 50 Gy or continued to 60 Gy if poor regression. The skin is allowed to heal and residual vulval tumor can be excised 4 weeks later if regression is incomplete. This would not apply to initially fixed or ulcerated groin nodes showing residual tumor; these areas require local booster doses. Excellent responses are frequently seen with this chemoradiation technique.

MORBIDITY FROM PELVIC RADIOTHERAPY

Acute side-effects

These mainly involve epithelial surfaces and occur during treatment.

1. The majority of patients experience mild diarrhea by the third week of pelvic radiotherapy. This is easily controlable with simple anti-diarrhea medication, advice on a low residue diet and avoidance of intestinal gas-producing foods.
2. Mild bladder irritability with frequency and dysuria may be experienced.
3. Skin reactions are unusual although obese patients may experience excoriation under skin folds and in the natal cleft. Advice given to patients include avoiding personal toiletries, tight clothing and washing the treated skin until 10 days have lapsed after the completion of treatment. A bland starch powder should be applied to the treatment area several times daily. Treatment should not be interrupted for mild skin reactions although wet desquamation may necessitate a rest period. Acriflavine emulsion or a steroid and local anesthetic cream may be applied to affected areas until healing occurs.

Late side-effects

These occur months to years after radiotherapy, involving slowly proliferating connective tissue, mainly the vasculature. Risk factors include large fraction size and high total radiation dose. Gradual vascular obliteration, replacement fibrosis and radionecrosis occur leading to stenosis, chronic ulceration or fistulation. Rectosigmoid complication include chronic diarrhea with or without the passage of fresh blood. Sigmoidoscopy should be performed to exclude other causes although biopsy should be avoided as healing in the affected area is poor. Mild occasional bleeding does not require any specific therapy although if patients are rendered anemic, Salazopyrin 1 g three times daily, steroid enemas and iron supplementation are used. Severe rectal bleeding with constant pain may require defunctioning colostomy, as would rectovaginal fistula or obstruction from sigmoid stenosis.

Small bowel

Obstructive episodes are difficult to manage because they involve one or more irradiated loops of ileum impacted in the pelvis due to previous surgery or pelvic inflammatory disease. Mild symptoms are managed with low residue diet and obstructive episodes are conservatively managed though persistent obstruction or an acute abdomen from perforation require laparotomy.

Bladder

Complications include contracture with small capacity, hematuria and vesicovaginal fistula. Ureteric obstruction leads to hydronephrosis with or without pain and is frequently a harbinger of pelvic recurrence rather that fibrotic obstruction. Treatment is individualized.

Ovarian ablation

This is inevitable and hormone replacement therapy should be offered to all premenopausal patients with cervical cancer undergoing pelvic radiotherapy. A combined preparation is preferable as occasionally patients experience withdrawal bleeds, indicative of residual functional endometrium.

Sexual counseling

This is imperative after radiotherapy and is detailed in Chapter 19.

CONSTRAINTS TO RADIOTHERAPY OF GYNECOLOGICAL CANCER IN DEVELOPING COUNTRIES

Patient factors

Cervical cancer is the most common malignancy in females in developing countries. The trend towards late presentation contributes to the high mortality. Reasons are absence of screening programs, lack of awareness of symptoms, unavailability of local medical facilities, delays from slow and inefficient referral patterns to the tertiary hospital/ oncology center.

Patients may also regard orthodox medicine as a last resort, often choosing to return home to consult the extended family and traditional healers.

Follow-up is often problematic, depriving patients of expert management of recurrent disease or treatment complications.

Personnel factors

It is estimated that in Sub-Saharan Africa there are only some 75 radiotherapists serving 285 million people. The situation with supporting staff required in a radiotherapy unit is equally critical.

In the future 'triaging' of patients with radical treatment for those considered curable and palliative treatment for others should be evaluated and training of personnel for radiotherapy units should be modified to provide for local disease profiles as has been instituted in Zimbabwe with WHO assistance.

17

Care of the terminally ill patient

L. Denny

INTRODUCTION

Despite significant advances in the modern management of gynecological malignancies, cancer remains a largely fatal disease. This is particularly true in developing countries where patients frequently present at an advanced or terminal stage of their disease.

Caring for women with advanced malignancy is a complex and often difficult process that requires a great deal of skill, attention to detail and appropriate yet active intervention.

The aim of management is the relief of suffering. Suffering in itself has many different components, both physical and emotional. Care of these patients requires attention to all aspects of personhood (Table 17.1). Modern technologic medicine with its emphasis on disease and its physical manifestations is an inadequate basis for terminal care. For example, morphine is an effective and reliable analgesic but it cannot treat the associated loneliness, alienation and depression that may accompany the experience of pain by an individual. Failure to address

Table 17.1 Components of Personhood

Personality/character
Culture
Life roles (social/work)
Relationships
Rights
Activities, habits, idiosyncrasies
Spiritual
Body
Loss of future
Family
Secret life
Past and accumulated life experience

the complexity of an individual's illness is all too often the cause of suboptimal care that exacerbates rather than relieves her suffering.

CLINICAL ASSESSMENT

Critical to effective terminal care is making the correct diagnoses with the realization that the clinical situation may change at any time.

The diagnostic steps are:

1. Ascertain the extent and nature or the neoplastic process with careful delineation of all involved systems.
2. Allow the patient to list her difficulties and ensure she determines her own priorities. It is tempting to project one's own perceptions onto the patient, with the risk that incorrect assumptions may be made. Listen to her subjective account and with careful questioning and concerned listening it should be possible to create a list of immediate and future concerns.
3. Determine the personal, social and cultural context in which the patient lives, including support networks, financial capability and other forms of healthcare the patient may be receiving, e.g. sangomas, spiritual healers, herbalists, homeopaths.
4. Ascertain the patient's own inner resources, for example how she has coped with crises previously. The diagnosis of cancer has been likened to a disaster and a patient's 'pre-disaster' resources arc an important indicator of how she will respond to the current crisis.
5. Contact the patient's personal system, which will usually be her immediate family but in some communities may involve consultation with the elders or the wider extended family. Not only will her wider 'system' provide potentially useful information but it will also give an indication of the extent of her social support. It is imperative, however, to obtain the patient's consent prior to consulting with other people. Do not further disempower an already ill and often powerless person.
6. Determine the patient's private and often unexpressed fears and expectations. These issues should be specifically addressed without either excessive optimism or pessimism.
7. Special investigations must be tailored towards the therapeutic value the information will provide.

DELINEATING THERAPEUTIC OPTIONS

In general the best terminal care relieves suffering with the least inconvenience to the patient or her family. It should facilitate freedom and independence without excessive and unnecessary hospitalization, medical investigation or invasive procedures. All treatment decisions and options should be carefully discussed with the patient and she should be the final arbiter. It is not possible to provide effective terminal care without the patient's participation in both decision making and the treatment itself.

PALLIATION

There are four components to effective palliation.

1. Specific anti-cancer therapies, e.g. palliative surgery, radio- or chemotherapy either to the primary lesion or to metastases.
2. Treatment of secondary problems related to the cancer, e.g. offensive infected vaginal discharges, excessive bleeding, paracentesis for malignant ascites, bowel obstruction (see below).
3. Recognition and correction of side-effects of anti-cancer therapy.
4. Treatment of conditions unrelated to the primary cancer, e.g. osteoporotic fractures.

Once therapy has been instituted it is essential to monitor its outcome and efficacy. New problems may evolve in the course of treatment and these may necessitate a change in management. The best judge of effective treatment is the well-informed patient and her family. Occasionally, however, it becomes necessary to impose one's views more forcibly, for instance with the patient who demands chemotherapy in the vain hope for cure, even though it is clearly not effective. This is one of the many ethical dilemmas encountered with terminal care and emphasizes the need for expert individualized care, preferably with a multidisciplinary team.

SYMPTOM RELIEF

Gynecological cancers tend to produce symptom complexes which are variable but nevertheless allow a degree of predictability and expectant management. These are listed in Table 17.2.

APPROACH TO MANAGEMENT OF PAIN

The principles of pain management are:

1. Reduce the pain stimulus.
2. Raise the pain threshold.

Table 17.2 Symptom complexes

Pelvic Mass syndromes with various manifestations of compression of vessels and organs, infiltration of nerves and ureters
Abdominal mass syndromes with alteration of bowel function and ascites
Perineal syndromes with ulceration and infection
Systemic disease with pleural effusions, metastases, metabolic disturbances due to renal failure, paraneoplastic syndromes
Treatment-related syndromes due to side-effects of radiation and/or chemotherapy

3. Characterize the pain and differentiate opioid sensitive from opioid insensitive pain.
4. Use the correct drug/s, in adequate dosage at the correct frequency and increase the dosage as the pain increases in intensity.

Reducing the pain stimulus

A careful and thorough history is the key to understanding the likely cause of the pain. Careful attention must be paid to adjuvant measures:

- Treating infection with local and systemic antibiotics
- The use of localized radiotherapy for bony metastases
- Neural blockade for nerve infiltration
- NSAIDs for associated inflammation
- Compression bandages and massage for painful lymphedema
- Surgical aspiration of compressive cystic pelvic masses.

Raise the pain threshold

It is important to differentiate the components of an individual's perception of pain and understanding the factors that aggravate the pain is critical. Factors that lower the pain threshold include:

1. Fear regarding the cause and meaning of the pain. For instance an explanation that the pain is due to sciatica rather than the cancer *per se* may make the pain more tolerable.
2. When pain is perceived to be out of control and overwhelming.
3. When pain is associated with anxiety, depression, loneliness, despair and alienation.
4. When the severity of the pain is in doubt.
5. With chronic pain.

Attention must be paid to adequate explanation and communication with the patient. Underlying depression and anxiety must be addressed both pharmacologically and with other therapies such as relaxation, psychotherapy and physiotherapy. If a patient has faith in non-orthodox forms of therapy this should be acknowledged and supported without the value judgement so common to western orthodox medical practice. Ideally, alternative therapies should be integrated into the management plan.

In addition, watching a loved one dying is invariably traumatic and if left unaddressed may well be an added source of distress and anguish. Simple explanation, acknowledging the emotional pain of the family and demonstrating care and concern may be sufficient to alleviate this frequently neglected aspect of terminal care.

Characterizing the pain

As a general rule of thumb opioid responsive and opioid non-responsive pain are equated with nocioceptive and non-nocioceptive pain. Nocioceptive pain responds to anti-nocioceptive measures, i.e. analgesics. Non-nocioceptive pain frequently does not respond to analgesic drugs in a predictable or reliable manner. The most typical examples are nerve damage and incident (movement related) pain. Other examples would be bladder and rectal tenesmus as well as perineal excoriation and ulceration.

Equally important pain syndromes are those occurring after chemo- and radiation therapy. Toxic peripheral neuropathies after vinca alkaloids or cisplatinum-based chemotherapy present with painful parasthesias and occasionally sensory and motor loss or autonomic dysfunction. Treatment consists of discontinuing the drug and the use of either tricyclic antidepressants or anticonvulsants such as carbamazepine. Pain usually resolves with resolution of the neuropathy.

Pain related to radiation is due to changes induced in the microvasculature of connective tissues surrounding peripheral nerve structures or fibrosis and chronic inflammation of tissues. Treatment may be difficult but resolution may be expected with time. The use of tricyclic antidepressants and anticonvulsants (as detailed above) as well as low dose corticosteroids (2–4 mg dexamethasone 8 hourly) should be considered.

Treating pain

Oral analgesic drug therapy is the cornerstone of managing cancer pain. WHO advocates a three-step ladder approach with the use of non-narcotic, narcotic and adjuvant analgesics, alone or in combinations, always titrated and adjusted to the needs of the individual. It is distressing that even today in the 1990s cancer pain is frequently undertreated due to the fear of inducing addiction and dependancy. It cannot be stated strongly enough that failure to adequately relieve pain is in essence negligent and unnecessary.

CLASSIFICATION OF ANALGESIC DRUGS

This is summarized in Table 17.3.

Mild analgesics

These are the first-line drugs. Their main limitation is that the analgesic efficacy has a ceiling effect, i.e. increasing the dose beyond a certain level does not produce additive analgesia. Paracetamol is equipotent with Aspirin in analgesic and antipyretic effects but has far less anti-inflammatory action.

The NSAIDs have analgesic effect equal to or greater than Aspirin and share the same adverse effects on the gastrointestinal, hematopoietic, hepatic and renal systems. NSAIDs differ in their pharmacokinetic profiles and it is essential to familiarize oneself with the half-life and duration of action of the particular drugs available for use.

Weak narcotics

Weak narcotics may be added to the drug regimen if non-narcotics are not effective. They provide enhanced analgesia by working

Table 17.3 Classification of analgesic drugs

Mild analgesics
– paracetamol
– aspirin
– NSAIDs (Non-steroidal anti-inflammatory drugs)
Weak Narcotics
– codeine
– oxycodone
– propoxyphene
Strong Narcotics
– morphine
– hydromorphine
– methadone
– meperidine

synergistically with the non-narcotic drugs. These drugs are usually present in fixed dose, commercially prepared mixtures with the problem that the dose of the admixed non-narcotic analgesic is often inadequate. It is essential to ensure that the full dose of aspirin (600–1200 mg per dose) or paracetamol (500–1000 mg per dose) is given in combination. Note also that these drugs have the same metabolism as morphine with similar side-effects of sedation and constipation if used in excessive dose. In addition, tolerance may occur.

Strong narcotics

Strong narcotics should be used to treat moderate to severe pain. Narcotic analgesics are capable of producing analgesia over a wide range of doses and do not have a ceiling effect to the analgesia, i.e. the greater the dose the greater the pain relief. It has been clearly shown that the two great fears about morphine, respiratory depression and drug dependence, do not occur when used to treat pain. If excessive sedation does occur it is an indication that the chosen dose is excessive for the pain experienced by the patient. The correct action is to reduce the dose, not to stop the drug.

Oral morphine has been labeled by WHO as an essential drug and is the preferred route of administration. Its oral bioavailability varies from 35 to 75%, its plasma half-life is 2–3 hours but its duration of analgesia is 4–6 hours. With repeated, regular administration the pharmacokinetics remain linear and the drug can be administered safely. Pain is much easier to prevent than to treat and it is essential to prescribe regular 4–6 hourly administration of the drug in order to prevent breakthrough or episodes of 'peak' pain.

Only if oral morphine is ineffective due to inadequate absorption should alternative routes be employed, including intramuscular, subcutaneous or intravenous. Rectal morphine is a reasonable alternative but absorption and therefore analgesic potential tends to be unpredictable.

SIDE-EFFECTS OF NARCOTIC AGENTS

There are a host of side-effects associated with the use of narcotic analgesics; the commonest are listed in Table 17.4.

1. Nausea and vomiting. This occurs in about 50% of patients but is variable in intensity and easily controled with conventional anti-emetics.

Table 17.4 Side-effects of narcotic agents

Nausea and vomiting
Constipation
Sedation
Confusion
Respiratory depression

2. Constipation. Constipation is an almost invariable side-effect due to a decrease in gastric secretions and peristalsis resulting in dry, hard stools. It is essential to prescribe concomitant laxatives and stool softeners with oral morphine.
3. Sedation. Sedation is frequent at the start of treatment but in the majority of patients improves or resolves within a few days. In elderly patients there may also be confusion and hallucinations which may necessitate a reduction in the dose. As a rule of thumb adverse effects with oral morphine are more likely in the absence of pain.

Other drug combinations

1. The use of steroids have been reported to reduce narcotic dosage requirements in terminal cancer patients with benefits far outweighing the potential risks. They have a particular role in reducing pain caused by bone metastases, spinal cord compression syndromes, raised intracranial pressure with headache and infiltration of peripheral nerves. Caution should be exercized in patients with known peptic ulceration and with diabetes.
2. Use of phenothiazines as adjuvant therapy in severe pain not adequately controled by morphine should be considered. Haloperidol 3–5 mg 8 hourly is a very useful additive as a co-analgesic and anxiolytic in a distressed patient.

GASTROINTESTINAL SYMPTOMS

The common GIT symptoms occurring in advanced gynecological cancer are listed in Table 17.5.

Nausea, with or without vomiting, may be induced by various pathways that include:

- Cortical pathways (anxiety related)
- Vestibular center (rich in histamine receptors)

Table 17.5 Gastrointestinal symptoms

Nausea and vomiting
Constipation
Abdominal cramps
Anorexia
Bowel obstruction
Bowel fistulae

- Chemosensitive trigger zone (CTZ) (rich in dopamine receptors)
- GIT due to gastric stasis, obstruction.

Nausea related to the CTZ (i.e. caused by drugs, uremia, hypercalcemia) requires a drug with high affinity for dopamine receptors such as haloperidol (3–5 mg, 8 hourly). If nausea is related to the GIT, gastrokinetic anti-nauseants such as metoclopramide (10–30 mg 8 hourly or 1 mg/kg 8 hourly) will promote gastric emptying and increase gut motility in the absence of bowel obstruction. Antihistamines (Phenergan 25 mg 8 hourly or Sparine 50 mg 8 hourly) may also be useful both for anti-nausea and anxiolytic effects. Prochlorperazine (25 mg 8 hourly per rectum or 5 mg 8 hourly orally) has both muscarinic and histamine receptor activity and is moderately useful although less specific. In addition, dexamethasone in low doses (4 mg three times daily) is effective in suppressing nausea as well as stimulating appetite.

MANAGEMENT OF INTESTINAL OBSTRUCTION

This is a common problem in advanced gynecological malignancy and may pose difficult therapeutic and ethical dilemmas.

For the first episode, conventional 'drip and suck' with nasogastric drainage and intravenous correction of fluid and electrolyte imbalance is a reasonable option. If the obstruction fails to settle in an otherwise systemically well patient, surgery should be considered. Surgical options include:

- Gastrostomy, ileostomy, colostomy
- By-pass procedures with primary anastomosis.

Clearly this is a difficult decision and requires careful balancing of benefit versus risk. The options should be fully discussed with the patient as well as the high risk of a recurrence especially if the obstruction is secondary to tumor rather than adhesions. Subjecting an already ill patient to a major surgical procedure may adversely affect the last days of her life with only very temporary relief of symptoms. On the other hand, if she is in reasonable health at the time surgery may dramatically improve the last weeks of life.

If conservative therapy fails and surgery is not a viable option alternative management includes:

1. Short course of oral or parenteral corticosteroids.
2. Hyoscine hydrobromide (25 mg 8 hourly) which acts as an anti-emetic as well as relaxing the gut and increasing the gut reservoir. Although the patient will vomit two to three times a day the frequency decreases as do the associated abdominal cramps. Used in conjunction with other anti-nauseants and minimal fluid intake (urine output plus 500 ml for insensible loss) may provide adequate relief of symptoms. Food should be restricted to blended highly refined 'baby-type' food.

MALIGNANT ASCITES

Malignant ascites is a common and distressing complication of advanced gynecological malignancy. Repeated paracentesis or the insertion of a drain with a one-way tap is the most effective treatment (Chapter 5). Diuretics should not be used.

ANOREXIA

Anorexia may be exacerbated by poor oral hygiene as well as oral fungal and other infections. Meticulous attention to mouth care is mandatory and may provide significant relief. In addition unpleasant odors from infected lower genital tract malignancies should be eliminated by frequent douching (dilute vinegar is as effective as the more expensive commercial antimicrobial preparations) and systemic and local antibiotics.

DIET

Manipulating diet may be of value and in general low residue soft foods should be advised, as for patients with bowel obstruction. Food supplements are useful but are very expensive and are not available in all settings. The emphasis should be on food of high nutritional value and the taking of frequent, small, easily digestible meals.

URINARY TRACT SYMPTOMS

Hydronephrosis with obstructive nephropathy and symptoms of pain and infection may require active management. The options are:

1. Palliative radiation to reduce tumor volume.
2. Percutaneous nephrostomies, especially where the home situation is such that the nephrostomies can be monitored without medical supervision. Occasionally as a temporary measure while administering radiation therapy.
3. Urinary diversion with ileal conduit. This is a major intervention and is a decision that should be taken with much care and thought, preferably by a multidisciplinary team (Chapter 5).
4. Treat the infection with no attempt to relieve the obstruction. Once the infection is treated a short course of dexamethasone may well temporarily restore ureteric patency.

FISTULAE

Rectovaginal (RVF) and vesicovaginal (VVF) fistulae, either as a consequence of the malignancy or radiation therapy, are a source of great distress and discomfort to patients. Major symptoms include:

- Offensive odors
- Pain due to excoriation and infection
- Constant soiling
- Isolation and embarassment.

Operative treatment in the terminally ill patient is rarely a viable option as major diversion procedures are required and even these procedures are not always effective. The best option is aggressive local cleansing combined with:

- Urinary antiseptics and alkalinization of the urine for VVFs
- Low residue diet with stool softeners for RVF
- Use of zinc ointments applied liberally to the perineum to protect against excoriation.

Local cleansing may be particularly difficult for patients who do not have access to running water and consideration should be given to hospitalization or local clinic care.

EDEMA

This may result from either lymphatic and/or venous obstruction and causes significant discomfort. There are no completely effective measures but the use of compression bandages, leg elevation and meticulous attention to prevention of trauma may provide some relief. Diuretics are not recommended.

CONCLUSIONS

An approach to various aspects of the management of patients with terminal cancer has been described. Central to the approach is understanding by patients, their families and physicians of the complexity of the process. Good palliative and terminal care demands careful attention to detail, perceptive and compassionate listening and often active intervention. The greatest sins in terminal care are to abandon patients with the comment that 'there is nothing more we can do for you', treating the disease rather than the person and not utilizing the patient's support system.

It has been clearly shown that the overwhelming majority of patients dying of cancer know the truth about their illness, whatever defences they employ to cope with their circumstances. Withholding information either at the request of the family or through one's own inability to impart bad news will add to the stress. Allowing patients to prepare themselves and their families for their impending death is an integral part of dying with dignity. Truthfulness combined with compassion is the patient's right and should never be withheld.

18

Traditional approach to the cancer patient

H. Zungu

Traditional healing was practised from time immemorial before the arrival of the settlers and missionaries for all kinds of diseases, cancer included.

Reference to tumors was found among the earliest Egyptian records in the period between 1500 and 2000 BC, and before the Exodus of the Jews from Egypt in the year 1513 BC cancer was treated by a corrosive paste administered on the body of the patient. This corrosive paste was not analyzed in detail by the ancient students of medicine because the medical knowledge of those physicians was purely empirical, largely magical and wholly unscientific.

The standard of practice used by traditional healers today is far better than that of the ancient traditional healers. A recently formed council oversees activities of these healers but prior to this, in the 1980s, a research project was undertaken by a few healers who came together with an idea of forming a council of healers and who traveled to East, West and Central Africa for 5 years to study various methods of traditional practice.

The patient after having been told at the clinic or hospital that she has cancer feels isolated and vulnerable, afraid of being hospitalized and being away from other members of her family. She will try all means of treatment no matter where it is found. She might first visit a traditional healer for alternative treatment and to clear her psychological turmoil about the strange disease affecting her. The main idea in visiting the traditional healer is to check whether the illness was caused by the wrath of her forefathers or if a spell has been cast against her by a sorcerer.

The healer is put to a test by the patient and expected to tell her why she has visited him before any treatment can start. The patient expects the healer to tell her about her past life and the present illness. During the discussion the healer must pause and get feedback from the patient as to whether she understands what is being said to her.

This is a type of religion to the patient like that practised by the ancient Israelites. When they were in trouble they approached their priests or prophets for their destiny. Kinsmen of the patient are as much concerned as the patient is about her future in regard to the new disease affecting her. The healer they visit should be one who is able to 'throw bones' and tell them about things that happened in the past and the present. The members of her family are very influential regarding her illness and treatment, no matter what the status of the patient, and she has to submit to her family's suggestions.

A properly trained traditional healer will always strive to keep a good reputation in the community. He will do this by not overcharging his patients and where he fails will accept personal limitations and hand over the continued care of the suffering one to those better equipped to continue treatment.

This action is in line with the ethics of the Traditional Healers' Council and refutes the statements made by those who are anti-traditional healers that patients under their care are not referred to orthodox medical facilities at an early stage.

The traditional healer will not at any time encourage the patient to discontinue the Western methods of treatment, even if the patient demands treatment. Instead she will be encouraged to complete the treatment from the orthodox medical practitioner. Western and traditional medicines cannot be applied simultaneously and even if the need may arise to undergo an operation a ritual will be pronounced to encourage the patient to face the operation with courage.

If the patient believes that cancer may end her life if not treated successfully, she will obey all the instructions given to her. She will visit the hospital or clinic on the dates set for her. If treatment is prolonged she will visit the traditional healer for alternative treatment.

The idea is not to promote competition between the orthodox medical doctor and the traditional healer but to act in a complementary way to help restore the patient's health. There still exists much doubt and mistrust in certain circles of orthodox medical doctors who reject tradition medicines out of hand and call it 'Mambo Jambo Taboo'. They cannot be blamed because they lack knowledge as to the role of a traditional healer in the community. They conclude that the training of traditional healers is not adequate because they expect it to fit into the Western concept. This will never happen.

The training of the three groups, who belong to the Traditional Healers' Council is as follows.

1. A traditional healer is commonly known as 'Nyanga' (one who heals with herbs) from teenage to adulthood. He must work under a well-trained Nyanga who has practical experience of not less than 5 years and will show him certain plants in the veld and explain their properties. Technical instruction such as grinding them into a fine powder, measurements and directions for use is given and when he has attained all this knowledge he must be referred to the local association of healers for a test before he can join their association. If he lacks knowledge in certain aspects he will be referred back for further training. If he succeeds he will be issued with the Association's Certificate. If that association is a member of the Traditional Healers' Council he will be further examined by the ethics and qualification committee of the Council.
2. The training of a 'Sangoma', a female diviner, and a male diviner an 'Isanusi' is different from that of the traditional healer initially although the end result is similar. Members of this group receive a calling from a forefather who wants them to do this type of work. It may begin with a constant dream or direction which will lead to visits to traditional healers for meanings and confirmation. If ignored it will result in ill health, which may appear in different ways such as delirium which may be confused with mental illness.

   The training will last for 1–2 years including several tests to prove the capability in divination. However, this is not the end of the training as now another course has to be completed including studying plants and their use under the guidance of an experienced healer. At the conclusion of the course another examination is set regarding plants and their use. A final certificate to practice will be issued only if the candidate is successful.
3. Finally there is the 'Herbalist, the medicine man'. The training is similar to that of the Nyanga traditional healer. He is expected to have a thorough knowledge of plants, their names and identification. He will keep a large amount of medicine (muti) in his shops and sell them to traditional healers, Sangomas and the public. He serves the public like a chemist and he can help a patient with minor ailments or mix certain herbs for a patient referred to him by a traditional healer. The main difference between the traditional healer and the herbalist is that the latter has no knowledge of bone throwing and the patient approaching him must explain his problems in order for him to mix appropriate herbs.

The healers accept the doctrine that God is the supreme being and the Provider of life in the universe and that all His laws must be obeyed.

The power of healing whether from the orthodox medical doctors or traditional healers derives from God, that is why each and every patient visiting the traditional healer must undergo ‘examination by bones’.

Traditional healers treat all people irrespective of race, color or creed and take a neutral stand as far as politics are concerned. They provide healthcare to the community impartially. The traditional healer can play an important role in the early detection of cancer in referring patients for Western treatment and encouraging them to continue treatment. Their understanding of the patients fears and cultural taboos make them ideal partners in managing the many psychological problems associated with cancer.

19

Psychosexual problems after cancer treatment

E. Sapire

Technical advances have resulted in dramatic improvements in the treatment and survival of patients with cancer and more attention is being given to their quality of life, with the focus changing from 'staying alive' to 'living'. Those who benefit from this progress must be helped to cope with the effects of surgery, radiation and chemotherapy. Once the crisis of survival has passed, the profound effects of mutilating surgery and radiation may threaten women whose self-image and femininity rely on their physical attributes. Their feeling of integrity as women may be shattered, especially if the effects on sexual organs disrupt sexual practices that brought pleasure and intimacy prior to the illness. The psychologic effects may be as disabling as the physical. Therefore the treatment aim should be as conservative as possible to obtain optimal therapeutic results with the least mutilation to genitalia possible.

The adverse psychologic, social and sexual disorders can be avoided or mitigated by awareness and sensitive counseling. This requires the recognition that people do not cease to be sexual because of age or illness even when that illness is cancer.

Their negative feelings about self-worth and sexuality can ultimately threaten their intimate relationship, as partners are driven apart and many mutually withdraw.

PRETREATMENT COUNSELING

This should involve both partners as neither should be left to handle these emotional and physical burdens alone. They should be informed about the physical and psychologic effects of the disease and treatment and about the counseling and support available. Information may have to be provided simply, patiently and repetitively. Explain the anatomy and the changes that will occur, the potential for sexual function after treatment and the need for hormone replacement therapy. Many opportunities must be given to the patient and her partner pre- and postoperatively to discuss their concerns separately and together.

It is important to acknowledge that the partner also experiences concerns. He may fear contagion or the effects of radiation and be concerned about his own sexual fulfilment. He may feel guilty about thinking about or feeling sexual while she is coping with the diagnosis and treatment of cancer or because she is so ill and he may fear causing pain. His stress and anxiety may be compounded by revulsion about her altered body. All these emotions can affect relationships and sexual interactions. Many problems can be prevented by discussing these issues. Most people accept that removal of cancerous tissue is necessary for recovery if this is clearly explained.

DURING CONVALESCENCE

Doctors must anticipate patients' anxiety about their sexuality whether they ask or not and make it easy for them to discuss their concerns. Patients may think it unseemly to raise this issue or assume that if nothing is said that sex can no longer be part of their lives. We must not render patients asexual because of our own embarrassment. Lack of concern or off-handed remarks can render a person permanently sexually disabled.

In the acute phase of illness, discussion about sex is clearly inappropriate but once the patient recovers it is necessary to provide clear information about what can be expected, whether it is necessary to abstain, when to resume and at what pace. It is important to be optimistic and reassuring but always honest and never raising false hopes.

It can be very helpful to talk to and share feelings with people who have undergone similar surgery and even to look at pictures of, for example, a stoma. After surgery both partners should look at the scar or bag in the supportive presence of the health professional. Before discharge from hospital both partners should be counseled about how to resume sexual activity and especially about the importance of maintaining intimacy and caressing during the period of healing.

Disease can be an alienating experience, the effects may be minor or devastating and can strengthen or destroy the relationship.

FACTORS THAT AFFECT SEXUAL FUNCTION

1. *Physical effects.* Any disease or treatment that interferes with innervation or the structure of the clitoris or vagina may make arousal and orgasm difficult. However, even after a pelvic

exenteration and removal of the vagina, labia and clitoris, some women have reported that they are still able to experience the sex response cycle.

The following symptoms may affect sexual responsivity in different ways: pain, debility, weakness, reduced energy, nausea, anorexia, fatigue, dyspareunia and reduced vaginal lubrication. Poor self-image may result in depression, can affect sexual responsivity and requires supportive counseling. These changes may be severe but are usually temporary.

Symptoms of estrogen deficiency will occur after radiotherapy or chemotherapy and include all menopausal symptoms. Adequate hormone replacement therapy is mandatory when not contraindicated.

2. *Psychologic effects.* Many women equate menstruation and fertility with femininity and their loss can affect sexual responsivity. Guilt may be linked to the diagnosis of genital cancer, possibly caused by previous sexual activity. Feelings of loss, sadness, frustration, resentment, anger and unattractiveness can interfere with sexual expression and behavior.

EFFECTS ON SEXUAL FUNCTION

Cancer of the cervix

It is important to deal with patients' feelings of guilt or shame, as some consider this diagnosis a punishment for excessive or casual sexual activity. Fear that continued sexual activity may cause recurrence, requires assurance.

Discussion before and after treatment should encourage women to resume coitus early to prevent the incapacitating vaginal changes that have been described. If possible, regular intercourse should take place once a week to maintain flexibility and patency of the vagina. Adequate foreplay and arousal is advisable before entry. Discomfort, vaginal bleeding and discharge may occur with contact during coitus but this is not evidence of recurrence of cancer. The side by side coital position is advised, as this allows the woman to control the degree of penetration. Where no partner is available the patient is advised to dilate the vagina manually or with dilators using KY jelly or estrogen cream.

Cancer of the vagina

The outlook for continued sexual function is poor. Dilators, lubricants and estrogen cream must be used after the operation to prevent stenosis.

Cancer of the vulva

Postoperative physical consequences of radical vulvectomy can be very troublesome. Deforming scars, vaginal stenosis, lymphedema and reduced movements of the lower limbs all occur. Altered body image plays an extremely important role and psychologic support is needed.

There are anecdotal reports of continued sexual function including orgasm even after clitoridectomy; however, 76% of women reported a worsening of their sex lives, 41% a deterioration in their emotional relationship with their partner, with a high incidence of hypochondriasis, depression and hysteria, 18% entered the psychotic scale. Psychologic and sex counseling are indicated.

Pelvic exenteration

This operation has gained acceptance for treating postradiation centrally recurrent gynecological malignancy. However, women who lose their vagina and clitoris can learn to explore and respond to stimulation of other erogenous zones such as the anus and scar tissue in the area of the vulva. They can attempt to improve their sensitivity to thigh, mouth and breast stimulation.

The most important factor in sexual rehabilitation is a partner who accepts the consequences of surgery and who continues to be interested in physical pleasure.

Counseling

Sexual function is not of primary importance when the patient's life is at stake. However, removal or mutilation of the vagina results in psychosomatic problems which can make social and sexual adjustment difficult, if not impossible. As the individual recovers from the surgical insult, the fear of persistent disease decreases. The patient begins to hope for complete recovery and concerns about psychosexual function emerge as a significant problem.

Counseling must be appropriate to the needs of the couple and not impose unwanted standards of sexual expression incompatible with their culture and norms. Where coital sex has been the only form of sexual expression, negotiation of cuddling and general pleasuring is often difficult, while negotiating autoeroticism, mutual masturbation, oral–genital and/or anal stimulation and the use of fantasy may be impossible. These options may become acceptable with sensitive counseling. Sexual assignments should be based on sensuality, tenderness and intimacy and less on performance and achievement with emphasis placed on body image and self-worth.

Specific suggestions

1. The use of lubricants and hormone replacement therapy when appropriate.
2. Positions. The woman-above position and 'L' or lateral position (with their bodies facing, at about 90 degrees, interlocking with the man's leg lowest on the bed) are comfortable. They allow the woman to control the depth of penetration during thrusting and to increase the sensation of depth for her partner by using her hand at the base of his penis.

SUMMARY

Gynecologists should be aware of the effects of the diagnosis of cancer and of treatment on patients' sexual function. Early involvement of the partner will reduce the psychologic impact of the illness on their sexual function. Their sexual well-being depends on their inner strengths, their attitude to sexuality and previous function. The health professional must inform them what to expect and discuss treatment options, fears about surgery, radiotherapy or chemotherapy. They must also be given several opportunities to discuss their concerns after treatment and should be counseled on extending their capacity to experience pleasure and intimacy and to show affection within the limitations of her illness.

In a developing country the following factors have to be taken into account:

1. Poor social conditions, housing with overcrowding, lack of privacy.
2. Illiteracy. Programs to educate patients in simple ways such as charts and comic books.
3. The ethnic and cultural norms of communities need clarification particularly in regard to sexual expectations.
4. Gender discrimination needs to be clarified. In many communities a patriarchal society ensures domination and subjugation of women.

Thus far only anecdotal evidence in regard to the above factors exists. In-depth research is necessary to serve these communities adequately.

20

Supportive measures for cancer sufferers

L. Greef

INTRODUCTION

> Medicine is not only a science, but also the art of letting our own individuality interact with the individuality of the patient.
>
> *Albert Schweitzer*

A comprehensive approach to the care of cancer patients requires the medical practitioner to be creative when offering choices to patients that will enhance their well-being. Knowledge of resources will enable the medical practitioner to decide what services would benefit individual patients and their specific circumstances.

Cancer touches the patient and the family at all levels of their being. Therefore we need to assist families in utilizing their innate ability to be part of the rehabilitation process and ultimately their own healing. Healing in this context not meaning being free of cancer but rather focusing on 'living' with cancer and not on 'dying' of cancer. Quality of life rather than quantity.

Cancer patients need to be seen as a part of a family system. A system that has the power to support and carry a patient through a crisis period. The emphasis therefore is on dealing with the cancer patient and the family as instruments that could assist in this healing process. This family involvement needs to be negotiated as early as possible, allowing members to be part of the treatment team and to guide and support each other.

HOLISTIC APPROACH

Within the medical model of dealing with cancer focus is often only on the physical aspects of the disease and its treatment. Practitioners tend to minimize the role of psychologic and spiritual components.

A holistic approach according to Lawrence Leshan needs to consider the following issues:

1. A patient exists on many levels that are equally important: physical, psychologic and spiritual.
2. All patients are unique, therefore a treatment program should be individualized.
3. A patient should be part of the decision-making team.
4. A patient has self-healing abilities that can aid the medical treatment program. Patients should be encouraged to explore the different avenues available to them.

By having a broader approach, health professionals can be creative and motivate and inspire patients and their families to become involved in their own rehabilitation process.

SERVICES AVAILABLE DURING DIFFERENT PHASES OF THE ILLNESS

Phase one: diagnosis

During this phase of the illness, the patient and family members are particularly vulnerable for suddenly their reality changes. The process of diagnosis is cumbersome and often frightening. Because of the uncertainty during this crisis time, the patient is often very lonely and fearful. They are overwhelmed by many new experiences and are intimidated by hospital procedures. Often they lack the assertiveness to reach out to medical staff for basic information.

During the diagnosis phase the patient has the need for information regarding:

- Illness
- Investigative procedures
- Possible treatment methods
- Implications of treatment
- Duration of treatment
- Prognosis
- Sources of this information
- Practical issues regarding treatment, e.g.
  - Where will treatment be given?
  - How often?
  - How to make appointments?
  - Will treatment be painful?

Who will administer treatment?
May a friend or family member accompany them to the treatment sessions?

The patient also has the following needs:

- To talk about the crisis
- To ask questions
- To know where and what resources are available
- To be treated as a whole person
- To know how to access emergency services within a bureaucratic structure
- To know the costs involved
- To know that they can ask for a second opinion
- To be part of the decision-making team
- To be actively involved in the treatment process complementing their medical treatment with one or more of the following avenues of help:
  Vitamins
  Minerals
  Exercise
  Diet
  Relaxation exercises
  Meditation
  Visualization
  Psychologic counseling
  Limited exercise program.

Phase two: treatment

The treatment of cancer is greatly feared because of the side-effects of the major treatment modalities.

It is of the utmost importance that the patient and the family are well informed concerning the treatment program which the medical team have recommended. If possible, patients should be given the choice of treatments accompanied by the relevant information in order to make an informed decision. This requires the medical practitioner to be sensitive to the needs of the patient and family, to be willing to spend time with the patient and to work through the treatment program and its consequences.

Honest discussion regarding the treatment's side-effects and the means of dealing with these side-effects is important. Linking the patient to supportive resources is essential, particularly if the medical staff are not available to support the patient and the family throughout this difficult period.

The treatment of cancer is often experienced by patients as a time of passivity when everybody is doing things to their bodies. They feel totally out of control and it is of great importance to foster a fighting spirit and a sense of personal control. This can often be accomplished by directing the patient towards psychologic counseling and other complementary helping strategies.

Needs of the patient during the treatment phase:

1. Need for information regarding different treatment options.
2. Need for information on side-effects of treatment on a general level.
3. Resources available to deal with side-effects on a medical level.
4. Practical assistance with issues like diet. This could be a means of contributing to the patients' own healing ability and give them a sense of control.
5. The patient needs time to question the treatment.
6. The patient reacts to treatment on an emotional level and these needs should be catered for. Early referral to a proper resource center will prevent unnecessary trauma and will assist in enhancing rehabilitation and healing by giving meaning to this crisis time.
7. Guidance with regards to exercize is needed as it might help the patient to stay active.
8. Involve the family during treatment procedures so that the patient is not isolated. This will also enhance the sharing process between patients and family members.
9. Encourage the patient to pursue complementary therapies if they have the need. These include progressive relaxation, meditation, visualization and imagery.
10. If treatment is by a medical professional in private practice, it must be remembered that a team approach is difficult to achieve. Special effort needs to be made to refer the patient to supportive services within the community. Similarly, the family will need these resources.
11. Children in these families require special consideration and referral for counseling before problems arise.
12. Practical problems are often a great stumbling block during treatment, for example:
    (a) Transport to and from treatment
    (b) Financial situation of families and availability of financial assistance

(c) Limited services in rural areas
(d) Lack of supportive family systems.

These problems need to be dealt with in order to ensure the patient's compliance to treatment.

Patients have a need for feedback about their test results and their meaning. Take time to discuss these with them.

CONCLUSIONS

The care of a cancer patient places severe strain on the medical and paramedical team members that care for them. If our goal remains to provide a comprehensive service, one that focuses on the patient's ability to live fully in the presence of cancer, we need to be aware of the variety of supportive services that are available.

Cancer patients and their families need all the help they can possibly get. Medical practitioners must take responsibility for developing their interpersonal skills in order to be sensitive to the needs of their patients on all levels of their existence, body, mind and spirit.

Further reading

Suggested booklist for cancer patients and their family members.

Penny Brohn, *Gentle Giants*, Century Hutchinson, 1987.
Stephanie Simonton, *The Healing Family*, Bantam Books, 1988.
Bernie Siegel, *Love, Medicine and Miracles*, Arrow Books, 1990.

General Information
Carl and Stephanie Simonton, *Getting Well Again*, Bantam Books, 1978, 1980, 1988 (3rd edn).
Sirkora and Heprey Smedley, *Cancer – What it is and how it is treated*, Basil Blackwell, 1985.

Personality and Stress related to cancer
Lawrence Le Shan, *You can Fight for Your Life*, Thorsons, 1980.

Complementary Approaches
Penny Brohn, *The Bristol Programme*, Century Hutchinson, 1987.

Index

Page numbers appearing in **bold** refer to figures and page numbers appearing in *italic* refer to tables.